THE END OF
CRAVING

Recovering the Lost
Wisdom of Eating Well

Mark Schatzker

AVID READER PRESS

New York   London   Toronto   Sydney   New Delhi

AVID READER PRESS
An Imprint of Simon & Schuster, Inc.
1230 Avenue of the Americas
New York, NY 10020

First Avid Reader Press hardcover edition November 2021

AVID READER PRESS and colophon are trademarks of Simon & Schuster, Inc.

For information about special discounts for bulk purchases, please contact Simon & Schuster Special Sales at 1-866-506-1949 or business@simonandschuster.com.

The Simon & Schuster Speakers Bureau can bring authors to your live event. For more information or to book an event contact the Simon & Schuster Speakers Bureau at 1-866-248-3049 or visit our website at www.simonspeakers.com.

Interior design by Carly Loman

Manufactured in Italy

10 9 8 7 6 5 4 3 2 1

Library of Congress Cataloging-in-Publication Data has been applied for.

ISBN 978-1-5011-9247-0
ISBN 978-1-5011-9249-4 (ebook)

For Greta, Violet, and Henry

CONTENTS

Introduction: The Mystery   1

Part I: One Disease, Two Cures

  1.   The New Road to Better Nutrition   15
  2.   The Old Italian Way   25

Part II: You Are a Metabolic Genius (and You Love It)

  3.   You're Hot. Then You're Not   37
  4.   The Quest for Pleasure   55
  5.   Too Much of a Good Thing   69

Part III: Nutritive Mismatch

  6.   How Sweet It Is   83
  7.   Not Losing Isn't Everything. It's the Only Thing   99
  8.   Creamfibre 7000   117

Part IV: The Help That Hurts

  9.   Why Does Food Taste Good, Anyway?   133
  10. You Are Eating Pig Feed   149

Part V: The Brain-Changing Power of Good Food

  11. The End of Craving   167
  12. Can This Be Fixed?   181
  13. A Visit to the Old Road   187

Acknowledgments   205
Bibliography   207
Notes   227
Index   245

The Mystery

The problem with mysteries is that most of the time they don't get solved, at least not the way we want. Life is not like the ending of a mystery novel, when the detective points at the murderer and says, "It was him." Mysteries are like Russian nesting dolls. You break one open only to find there is another smaller, harder question waiting for you inside. And the game continues.

On a sunny September day in 2014, in the Jasmine Room at the DoubleTree hotel in Bethesda, Maryland, the mystery was food. There are many mysteries when it comes to food, but this was the big one, a nutritional debate that had been raging for decades: What makes people gain weight, carbs or fat? A scientist named Kevin Hall, from the National Institutes of Health, was standing at the lectern advancing slides in PowerPoint, preparing to deliver the answer.

Over the past several months seventeen overweight or obese men had participated in a study of the controlled, scientific feeding of carbohydrates. Each and every day, they ingested an average of 2,398 calories, 48 percent of which were from carbohydrates and 36 percent from fat. The men were not permitted to leave so much as a crumb. If they received guests, they conducted their visits in full public view to ensure that no food, not even gum, was secretly shared. There were no conjugal visits. Two days a week were spent in a metabolic chamber, a high-tech room outfitted to measure how much oxygen the men consumed and how much carbon dioxide they released—it even tracked their movement with radar. For twenty-eight days the men ate, watched TV, used a stationary bicycle, went to the bathroom, and slept.

Then they did it all over again for another twenty-eight days—only now they were in the high-fat or "ketogenic" phase. The second diet was almost identical to the first, with the same number of calories and the same amount of protein. But there was an important difference: fat and carbs had swapped roles. Now 77 percent of the calories came from fat and a mere 6 percent from carbs. All the while, Kevin Hall and his team collected blood and urine samples and analyzed every available point of data so that they could, once and for all, settle the great carbs-or-fat debate.

IT IS a debate that stretches back at least as far as 1972, with the publication of *Dr. Atkins' Diet Revolution: The High Calorie Way to Stay Thin Forever*, one of the most influential diet books of all time. Humans, Dr. Atkins argued, had naturally evolved to eat meat but were being fed carbohydrates, to which they were "allergic," and which made them accumulate fat. His advice was simple: stop eating bread and cereal and drinking fruit juice. Instead, eat more of what humans were meant to consume: cheese, eggs, and meat.

Dr. Atkins, alas, was twenty years too early to his own party. In 1977, the American government released *Dietary Goals for the United States*, a document that urged the nation to "increase carbohydrate consumption" and cut down on butterfat, eggs, and red meat. Atkins's anti-carb message was quickly drowned out by a growing national crusade against fat. Americans became ever more sure that everything wrong with their diet was all the fault of this single nutritional villain. Why did people get fat? Because they ate fat. So Americans declared war on nature's most calorically potent macronutrient. Diet salad dressings were poured on iceberg lettuce. Sandwiches were made with low-fat mayonnaise, lean slices of turkey breast, and low-fat cheese. At dinner, skinless breast of chicken was served next to a mound of steamed rice and boiled vegetables. At brunch, the true nutrition sophisticates asked that the omelet please be made from egg whites.

It was all a mammoth failure. Despite all those lean, hard-fought years of avoiding fat, the nation got fatter. All that supposedly healthy food didn't reduce obesity—it pushed the national rate up by fifteen points. More than two decades after Dr. Atkins sounded the alarm against carbohydrates, America was finally ready to take his advice.

Almost overnight, meat was back. Guests would show up to dinner parties and refuse the salad, refuse the garlic bread, and refuse the potatoes, but help themselves to three portions of flank steak. Around the watercooler, coworkers shared stories of the crippling carb cravings and heinous farting that accompanied the miracle of high-fat weight loss.

In 2002, a science writer named Gary Taubes published a sensationally popular article in the *New York Times Magazine* called "What If It's All Been a Big Fat Lie?" In it, he articulated what would become the leading dietary theme of a generation: "It's not the fat that makes us fat, but the carbohydrates, and if we eat less carbohydrates we will lose weight and live longer." Taubes would go on to publish several deeply researched books as more scientists and doctors joined the anti-carb camp. What had started as a too-good-to-be-true fad diet featuring unlimited bacon was beginning to seem as if it might work. The country's love of bread, pasta, rice, chips, doughnuts, fruit juice, and soft drinks came to seem like nutritional suicide. Taubes even introduced America to the hormone at the root of the problem.

Insulin regulates energy metabolism. When we eat, insulin is secreted, which sends the sugar and fat we consume into cells to be stored. Between meals, as insulin levels drop, these stored fuels are gradually released back into the bloodstream. According to the "carbohydrate-insulin model," as it would come to be known, a diet rich in carbohydrates, especially refined carbohydrates, produces excessively large secretions of insulin. This not only lowers blood sugar levels, it promotes the uptake of fat into fat tissue and also inhibits fat from being released into the blood to be used as fuel. What follows is a state of "internal starvation," leading to a reduction in energy expenditure, which we experience as lethargy, along with an increase in hunger. The now ravenous eater consumes another heaping portion of carbs, which causes another excessive burst of insulin, and the whole abysmal cycle— hunger, carbs, insulin, lethargy, hunger, carbs, insulin—plays out again. Obesity, according to this model, is simply a carbohydrate-induced metabolic defect that causes too much fuel to be stored and not enough to be used.

At long last, America had discovered the true cause of its dysfunctional relationship with food. Fat wasn't making people gain weight. Carbs were the problem all along.

In 2009, Gary Taubes visited the National Institutes of Health to give a talk on the carbohydrate-insulin model. Kevin Hall was in the audience. Hall was an agnostic when it came to the carbs-versus-fat debate. His PhD was in physics, and he was developing a complex mathematical model of human metabolism. But Taubes's argument had a compelling logic. If the human body is capable of using both fat and carbohydrates as fuel, it seemed reasonable that one might have a metabolic advantage over the other. A couple of years later, Hall proposed doing a rigorous study in which subjects were kept in a hospital setting and fed each diet while researchers measured precisely how the energy was being burned. Taubes was game. He had recently formed a nonprofit called the Nutrition Science Initiative (NuSI), which had received millions of dollars in funding.

Now, NEARLY half a century after Dr. Robert Atkins freed the low-carb genie from the bottle, the results were in. Standing at the Jasmine Room lectern, Kevin Hall advanced the slides.

Some of the data looked good. The high-fat diet resulted in a whopping 50 percent drop in insulin secretion—just what the anti-carb camp predicted. Within hours of being put on the low-carb diet, the subjects began burning more calories—again, just what the carbohydrate-insulin hypothesis predicted.

But, that spike of calorie burning was tiny, just a hundred calories per day, nowhere close to the hundreds of calories that had been predicted. Then, the data just got ugly. According to the carbohydrate-insulin model, the subjects were supposed to lose more fat during the low-carb phase, but the experiment's results indicated just the opposite—they lost fat faster on the high-carb diet. Carbs, it turned out, were better than fat. But only an itty bit better—the advantage was so small as to be academic. It was, however, most definitely not what the carbohydrate-insulin model predicted.

To Kevin Hall, what stood out most about these two diets wasn't their differences; it was their similarities. Here were two chemically different fuels—one sweet and starchy, the other oily and gooey—and the human body possessed a stunning talent to utilize each equally well. "It would be like filling your car with either diesel or regular gasoline," Hall explains, "and barely noticing a difference."

Taubes saw things differently. He thought Hall had bungled the experimental design and that the data were inconclusive. The mood in the Jasmine Room was, to put it lightly, tense. Hall remembers Taubes saying, "You've done a very good job of shooting this model in the leg, but you haven't killed it."

The now-wounded carbohydrate-insulin model limped into another fat-carb study, a massive $8 million endeavor at Stanford run by a highly respected researcher named Christopher Gardner. This experiment wasn't conducted in some laboratory outfitted with radar where people had to hand over their urine. It took place in the real world, with real people going about their lives as they normally would. Instead of seventeen participants, there were more than six hundred. For an entire year, half ate a healthy low-carb diet and the other half ate a healthy low-fat diet. If cutting carbs truly was easier than cutting fat, surely this experiment would show it. And if low-fat diets caused a metabolic defect that causes weight gain, surely this experiment would show it.

The results were, once again, amazing. And once again, it wasn't the differences between the two diets that stood out—it was the similarities. Both groups, on average, lost about the same amount of weight. They consumed the same number of calories, the same amount of protein, and secreted similar spurts of insulin. Even the range of success within the groups was, as Christopher Gardner puts it, "stunningly similar." In the low-fat group, a handful of individuals lost serious weight—sixty pounds or more. It was the same in the low-carb group. A small number of ill-fated participants in the low-carb group somehow managed to *gain* more than twenty pounds, despite their participation in a weight loss study. Same in the low-fat group. If you looked at a graph of weight loss for each set, they appeared as similar as identical twins.

There have now been dozens of controlled feeding experiments that have pitted fat versus carbs on human subjects numbering in the hundreds. Some give the advantage to fat. A few more give the advantage to carbohydrates. But the advantage, if there is one, is small. The stunning similarity of these two nutrients is no longer stunning.

So, mystery solved. The most ascendant theory of weight gain of the past twenty-five years—that eating too many carbohydrates causes overweight and obesity—is wrong.

WHICH JUST leaves us with more mysteries. For instance, what happened during the 1980s? As the research demonstrates, a human being can lose weight on a low-fat diet. Yet, when America attempted to do just that, the country collectively put on weight. As we all now are aware, Americans truly overdid it on the carbs. But they couldn't even get the "low-fat" part right. Despite the low-fat dressings, skinless chicken breasts, and ultralean hamburger patties that taste like burnt hair, America's fat intake did not go down. It stayed even. Despite this enormous, countrywide effort to eat less fat, Americans could not eat less fat.

What happened next is even more baffling. Due to the success and popularity of the anti-carb movement, Americans reduced their annual consumption of wheat by about fifteen pounds per person. Since 1999, consumption of sugar has dropped from forty-seven teaspoons per day to thirty-eight. It all sounds like good news—yet, in that same period, the rate of obesity has climbed from 31 percent of the population to more than 42 percent. It doesn't seem to matter what we stop eating; we find something else to eat and keep gaining weight. It is as though some force, some invisible hand, is compelling people to put food in their mouths.

Forty-seven scientists and doctors from some of the world's top research institutions encountered that same invisible diet-ruining force when they undertook an enormous, extremely expensive study called the Women's Health Initiative Dietary Modification Trial in 1993. Their goal was to see if it was possible to reduce strokes and heart attacks in postmenopausal women by getting them to eat less fat and more fruits, vegetables, and grains. The endeavor was of epic proportions, with nearly fifty thousand women involved. They took part in eighteen "behavioral modification" sessions led by certified nutritionists during the first year and met four times a year thereafter. All throughout, each woman received personal feedback and targeted messaging by phone or mail. Science would, at long last, come to know if eating more apples and oatmeal and less mayonnaise would reduce the risk of cardiovascular disease in postmenopausal women.

Except they never quite got the answer. Despite the meetings, the phone calls, and the millions of dollars spent, modifying the diets of these many women seemed to be impossible. Fat intake went down but then crept back up. Fruit and vegetable intake reached its goal of at least five servings a day, then slipped. Grain intake didn't budge. As an editorial in the *Journal of the American Medical Association* glumly put it, the "achieved dietary levels fell short of goal."

This outcome is anything but unique. Even when people are able to muster the will to eat less, they fail. A few years ago, a group of scientists at Yale University set out to see if posting calorie information next to restaurant menu items could help people eat more sensibly. Seeing those numbers, it turned out, had a measurable and positive effect on food choices—people chose smaller portions and ate less than the group that didn't see the calorie numbers. But it didn't last. The calorie counters would go home and eat dinner or have a snack in front of the TV, and by the end of the day half of them had consumed just as many calories as the group that never saw the calorie counts. In 2008, New York City passed a law requiring fast-food restaurants to post calorie labels on their menus. Customers reported not only that they saw these labels but used the information to reduce the amount of calories they consumed. Yet, five years after the law was passed, the average number of calories ordered had gone up instead of down.

Every year, millions of men and women all over the world make a heartfelt and concerted effort to eat less food. Like a freshly hatched salmon fry whose life goal is to return to the river of its birth, they face crushingly bad odds. They lose weight at first. But the weight comes back, usually starting around the six-month mark. The exasperated dieter swears he is eating less, but the scale claims otherwise. As many as two-thirds will eventually regain more weight than was initially lost.

When it comes to dieting, the real surprise are those that succeed, the tiny percentage of people who lose a great deal of weight—thirty pounds or more—and keep it off. It is a life-consuming effort. Many get divorced, move to a new neighborhood, or to a different city altogether. Their days are marked by weight-loss rituals: breakfast is obligatory, weigh-ins occur sometimes several times a day, and desserts are permitted only on weekends. A startling number of these people become dietitians. Achieving serious and lasting weight loss is like becoming a religious convert and joining the FBI's witness protection program all at the same time.

IMAGINE YOU walked into a room and found two people arguing about the cause of the common cold. One insists colds are caused by coughing. The other passionately argues that the sniffles are the root.

This is how we see our food problem. We believe eating too much food is the cause of obesity, when, in fact—like a runny nose or a cough—it is a symptom of something deeper, something nearly invisible. For decades now, we have been searching, fruitlessly, to find a way to get people to eat less. It is time to ask a different question: Why would someone consume food to the point of ill health and, eventually, death?

It was not always this way. Something happened. Some change took place in the world that is causing people—hundreds of millions of people—to set out on a deranged hunt for too much food. That change, whatever it is, took place within the last several decades.

This book is an attempt to find the answer. It will not lay the blame at the doorstep of a single nutrient, nor will it tell you there is a secret and easy cure. It will argue, rather, that our dysfunctional relationship with food stems from a fundamental and all-powerful myth, which is that humans are constitutionally primitive and dim-witted when it comes to eating. We believe evolution has designed us to be fat and that our natural urges are so out of touch with our actual nutritional requirements that not only do we suppress and abhor these basic impulses, we chemically alter food to lessen the damage it inflicts. When it comes to eating, we view ourselves as helpless slaves to pleasure who can only be saved by science.

The truth is that the brain is a more intelligent eater than we are capable of comprehending. It is one of evolution's great masterworks, informed by an unfathomably complex network of sensors, nerves, hormones, and chemical messengers. The brain achieves a level of nutritional precision that is stupefyingly exact. It can anticipate food shortages and can eat its way out of sickness. It even changes physics—butter floats in water, but in the human mouth, it tastes heavy, because the brain understands that butter is rich in calories while water has none.

This is the crux of the problem. We are so certain that food itself is to blame that for nearly a hundred years we have been attempting to fix what nature has gotten so badly wrong. The result is that, molecule by molecule and additive by additive, food has become a strange imitation of itself. The harder we fight to correct the defects of nature, the worse things get. The magnitude of the failure would be astounding if it were not so tragic.

Obesity is a sickness. People suffer because of it, and they die because of it. But obesity is also a normal reaction to the changes we have inflicted upon food. Our attempts to "improve" food have achieved the opposite effect. By trying to fix what was never wrong in the first place, we have produced the perfect conditions for obesity. People do not eat too much because they are lazy, self-indulgent, or weak. They eat because they want to. They are tormented by a desire, a craving—a force—that springs from the very core of their being.

This is the story about what happened to food and what happened to us, and about how we might begin to think about fixing a problem we are only now beginning to understand.

PART I

One Disease, Two Cures

1

The New Road to Better Nutrition

In the fall of 1786, the most famous writer in German history was experiencing a midlife crisis. Johann von Goethe was bored and irritable, his creative output had stalled, and he was on the cusp of breaking off an intense yet nonsexual ten-year affair with a beautiful woman who was married to a powerful bureaucrat. At three in the morning on the third day of September, Goethe crept out of bed, hopped quietly into a horse and buggy, and left the life he knew behind him.

Traveling under a fake name, he headed east, then turned south and crossed the Alps. On the ninth day, he reached the town of Rovereto, where the language switched to Italian. Three days after that, as he was setting out toward Venice, he noticed something odd about the locals. The women, he wrote in his diary, appeared pale. Their skin was sallow and had an odd brownish cast. The children, he added, "looked equally miserable."

The malady had a name: *la pellagra*, which meant "rough skin" in the local dialect. What the German traveler could not have realized is that he was witnessing the beginnings of a brutal epidemic, one that would last more than a century and kill hundreds of thousands of people. The symptoms would appear every year around the middle of April. A farmer—it always started with farmers—would notice a dark red spot on the back of his hand, which would fade, leaving a gleaming, scaly patch. A year later, the spot would return, this time bigger and darker. The spots would start spreading, first to the legs and then the feet. The farmer would begin to drool, his gums would bleed, his teeth would fall out. Wracked with bloody diarrhea, he would stop eating. In the most severe cases, neurological symptoms would develop— namely dizziness, delirium, motor disorders. Victims could be found doing the strangest things. Some would set off wandering. Others ate dirt or attacked children. A shoemaker from a village north of Venice sliced off his penis and threw it out the window.

Farmers were not pellagra's only victims. Women suffered more severely than men, and in greater numbers. In time, northern Italy would become dotted with pellagra "asylums," their halls filled with sisters and mothers and daughters, bone thin, their skin brown and scaled.

What was the cause of this terrible disease? No one knew. Some believed it was a "sickness of the poor." While this made a little bit of sense—rich people never got pellagra—there were parts of southern Italy that were even poorer than the poorest districts of the north, and they remained untouched by the disease. Other theories ran the gamut: pellagra was an animal disease that had jumped over to humans. It was caused by dust that penetrates the skin. It was a liver disorder. It was caused by the sun, rotten food, imperfect digestion, a lack of salt, foul water, aluminum salts. One scientist even proclaimed that pellagra was the product of spores that get in the blood, where they spontaneously burst into flame.

Whatever the cause, "rough skin" could not be stopped. A hundred years after Johann von Goethe wrote about those sickly looking women in his diary, more than 104,000 Italians would fall prey to the disease, and a cure was nowhere in sight.

IN 1902, a Georgia farmer with a bad case of hookworm paid a visit to his doctor. The patient's hands and legs, the doctor wrote in a report, were covered in blisters. The sores appeared in spring and had for the past fifteen years, at which point the farmer would lose his appetite and have fantasies of killing himself.

Pellagra had come to the United States.

By 1906, pellagra had spread to Alabama; it was in Texas the year following, and within two years reached the Carolinas, Mississippi, Arkansas, Virginia, Tennessee, and Illinois. Entire towns succumbed. In Italy, pellagra clung to the north, but in the United States, it made its home in the South, which became known as the Pellagra Belt.

American scientists were as stumped as their Italian counterparts, and even the dimmest statistical flicker would be seized upon as evidence of cause. Pellagra, some theorized, bore some kind of relation to water. People living two hundred to five hundred yards from a river, it was observed, were more susceptible to the condition than those who lived close or far away. Jews never got pellagra. Neither did divorcées, but being married, for some unknown reason, substantially increased risk.

Other scientists believed pellagra was an infection that thrived in the hot, humid South. An outbreak at the Mount Vernon Hospital for the Colored Insane, in Alabama, appeared to confirm the hypothesis. Patients entered the hospital in good health, only to fall ill. The healthy patients, it seemed obvious, were catching pellagra from the sick ones.

More experiments were conducted. In 1913, a scientist in New Orleans harvested skin, intestines, and other body parts from a dead pellagra victim and injected them into two monkeys. Both appeared to contract pellagra, and one monkey died. A different team of scientists repeated the experiment with seventy-seven rhesus monkeys, two Java monkeys, and three female baboons. Not a single one died from pellagra.

Some scientists outright rejected the infection theory. They were certain pellagra was caused by a parasite, one that was carried by insects. But even within this faction there was disagreement: one camp believed sand flies were the carrier, while another claimed it was mosquitoes. Amid all the raging disagreement, pellagra raged on.

In 1914, the surgeon general dispatched a top expert in infectious diseases to the Pellagra Belt. Dr. Joseph Goldberger, a Hungarian-born Jew from New York City, arrived at an orphanage in Jackson, Mississippi, where 172 children had been diagnosed. To anyone who knew anything about infectious diseases, the New York City expert appeared at best confused and at worst terribly ill-informed. The hygienic and sanitary conditions at these orphanages were appalling—a breeding ground for bacteria—and yet Goldberger explicitly instructed staff not to change a thing. Instead, he put the orphans on a peculiar diet of buttermilk, eggs, peas, and beans. Even stranger, it seemed to work. By the next spring, only one patient had relapsed. At a sanatorium in Georgia, Goldberger and his magic diet brought the number of pellagra cases from seventy-two down to zero.

What Goldberger did next was yet more odd: he attempted to *create* pellagra. In 1915, twelve convicts in a Mississippi prison were offered a deal: if they agreed to adhere to a diet of Goldberger's choosing for six months, they would be freed. Day after day, week after week, the Pellagra Squad, as they became known, dined on a relentless regimen of biscuits, "mush," rice, cane syrup, coffee, a "gravy" made from pork fat and flour, and sugar. By the end of the experiment, six of the convicts had pellagra.

The medical establishment had it all wrong, Goldberger declared. Pellagra was not infectious and was not an infection—it was a dietary disorder. Local experts, however, dismissed the stranger from New York City. Goldberger's experiment was derided as "half baked" by a prominent Birmingham physician, and his research was savaged in a long and bizarre article published in the *Journal of the American Medical Association* that passionately argued that Goldberger's theory was based on a misunderstanding of the scrotum. Determined to prove his critics wrong, Goldberger organized what would come to be known as "filth parties." He extracted blood from pellagra victims and injected it into sixteen volunteers, including himself and his wife. Not a single person fell victim to the disease. He scraped off skin scales and collected pellagra urine and diarrhea, blending it with flour and kneading it into a dough, which he fed it to his wife and the other volunteers. No one got pellagra.

As the 1920s drew to a close, the truth had become undeniable. Pellagra wasn't a disease; it was a form of starvation. There was a microscopic substance essential for the continuation of life that was only found in foods such as milk, beans, and meat. Without it, the body started falling apart. It began with blisters, progressed to diarrhea, wandering, and confusion, and ended with death.

Pellagra thrived in the South because Southern sharecroppers planted cotton "from fence post to fence post." With their meager earnings, they bought food at the local grocery store or commissary, which, like the land they worked, was often owned by their landlord. The poorest could afford a diet no better than what Goldberger fed the Pellagra Squad, an endless rotation of pork fat, molasses, and grits that lacked essential substances necessary to keep them healthy.

It was a world-changing revelation. Food wasn't just what you put in your mouth; it was a highly complex substance made up of tiny, often inscrutable pieces. The microscopic substances that worked to keep the body running, we know now, are vitamins. And the vitamin whose absence causes "rough skin" would come to be called niacin, also known as vitamin B_3.

If corn, molasses, and pork fat is all there is to eat, you get sick and you die. If you were a woman of reproductive age, and your body produced hormones that affected niacin metabolism, or what precious little niacin you had was being drained out of your body in breast milk to nourish your infant, the risk of getting the disease was much greater.

Pellagra was the result of a lethal blend of poverty and geography. Corn was cheap and Southerners were poor. In the opening decades of the twentieth century, pellagra killed more than one hundred thousand Americans.

NOW THAT pellagra's cause had been identified, the next question was how to stop it. Yeast was one solution. In the spring of 1927, a doctor named William DeKleine fed yeast mixed with water to a young black woman who was described as "a bag of bones at the end of pellagra's final starvation." Two weeks later, the doctor returned to find his eighteen-year-old patient bright-eyed and upright, her sores all healed. Liver was another cure. If you fed it to "pellagrins," they returned to good health as though by magic. Some common thing, some substance in both liver and yeast, was the key to this mystery.

A scientist at the University of Wisconsin named Conrad Elvehjem set out to isolate this antipellagra substance by extracting every single chemical from liver. One of them was nicotinic acid, a chemical that had been used for years to develop photographs. When nicotinic acid was fed to dogs sick with pellagra, they sprang back to good health. Joseph Goldberger's pellagra-preventing substance had been found. The world had its newest vitamin.

A year later, scientists began treating pellagra victims with nicotinic acid, which is now understood to be a form of niacin. It was a scientific miracle. When the sick were fed pure nicotinic acid, they felt a flush of warmth, and a glow of health swept over them. Their skin tingled as though they could feel the vitamin replenishing each little cell.

Yet this cure, however miraculous, still did not solve the country's pellagra problem. The government could not conscript an army of nurses to patrol the rural South, feeding sick mothers yeast or sticking niacin-filled syringes into suicidal farmers. It was becoming more obvious that the real problem went far deeper: food and people. Food, by nature, was nutritionally imperfect—lacking in substances vital to life. And people had no idea what was good for them and what wasn't.

In 1941, the US government decided to take action and rid itself of the pellagra problem once and for all. It officially encouraged the addition of niacin to white flour, along with thiamin, another recently discovered vitamin, and iron. Two years later, a third vitamin, riboflavin, was added to the mix. White flour, which had for so long delivered nothing more than nutritionally empty carbs was now "enriched." The FDA later added pasta to the list of nutritionally improved foods, followed by white rice, cornmeal, and grits. By the end of the decade, more and more states made enrichment—the nutritional fortification of empty carbs— the law of the land. The effect was magnificent. When Mississippi passed its fortification legislation, cases of pellagra plummeted from 101 per hundred thousand to fewer than 1 in a single year.

Poof! America's pellagra problem was gone.

Fortification was fast, simple, and amazing. With a dusting of a few chemicals, the nutritional flaws in food were corrected. Untold doses of vitamins now started entering people's cells via foods as innocuous as toast and doughnuts. Now you could eat all the grits you wanted; there was no way you'd get pellagra. It was, arguably, America's greatest-ever triumph of nutritional science and public health. Not only did it cure thousands, it offered a glimpse of a glorious century that lay ahead, one fueled by twin engines of science and industry.

ENRICHMENT MAY have rid the South of pellagra, but it is just one chapter in a longer and more tragic story. What seemed like a resounding victory turned out to be more like a temporary reprieve. The South's disease of poor nutrition did not disappear, it just changed forms. A century ago, thousands of people were covered in skin scales. Today, they have bodies that are, by the standard of "normal," misshapen; their cells respond abnormally to one of the most important hormones in vertebrate physiology: insulin. Jackson, Mississippi, where Joseph Goldberger cured sick orphans, is now one of the fattest cities in America.

You won't find any cases of pellagra, but you will find more than fifteen clinics that offer obesity treatment in a city of less than two hundred thousand. Today, the Pellagra Belt is called the Obesity Belt—a raging zone of ill-health that stretches from the Gulf states north towards Pennsylvania.

Of the two epidemics, obesity is by far the worst. It kills three times as many people in a single year as pellagra did in forty. Like pellagra, obesity disproportionately affects the South, the poor, women, and blacks. Its victims are shunned and seen as objects of contempt, as though the disease signifies a fault of character.

And just like pellagra, the disease features a revolving cast of experts, each with a different cure. Besides fat and carbs, scientific theories of weight gain have included television, cars, escalators, video games, supermarkets, a lack of supermarkets, "obesogenic chemicals," stress, artificial lighting, not enough sleep, and air-conditioning.

It is one of history's most painful ironies. In the last hundred years, we have learned to cure certain cancers and have prevented untold millions of heart attacks. We can take an organ from a dead person and implant it into a living person. But food—the nourishment we require in order to live—bedevils us. If the history of the South tells us anything, it would seem to be this: there is no winning when it comes to food. We solved one mystery only to find ourselves confounded by another.

2

The Old Italian Way

But just think of how bad things could have turned out. For example, consider Italy's response to pellagra, which was archaic almost to the point of comedy. The Italian government didn't dispatch doctors to the countryside bearing yeast or niacin. It didn't add vitamins to its death-inducing polenta. It called, instead, for bread to be baked in communal ovens. The government encouraged the poor they ought to raise rabbits, because rabbit meat was cheap. Even wine, of all things, played a role in Italy's battle against pellagra, and it actually helped, not that anyone had any clue as to why. (It was because the poorly filtered wines of the day were clouded with yeast, which, as scientists would later learn, is a rich source of niacin.)

Bunny rabbits, bread, and *vino*. It was as though the king had placed his half-wit nephew in charge of health policy. Across the Atlantic, America was embarking on its sunny new road to health and vitality, a route lit by the discoveries of modern science. Italy, by comparison, was like some stubborn peasant that preferred to stick to the path it knew, the old road.

Yet, that old road turned out to be a good one. It led Italy out of pellagra, albeit more slowly. In 1899, there were close to 73,000 cases of pellagra. After the government passed laws promoting rabbit meat and communal bread, it fell to 55,000. By 1920, there were just 202 cases of pellagra in what had once been its pulsating epicenter, Veneto, and seven years later, the Fascist dictator Benito Mussolini declared the pellagra epidemic was no more. Today, the disease is as rare in northern Italy as it is the American South. The country famous for its food somehow ate its way out of a crippling epidemic.

Here is another surprise. When it comes to eating and health, things are still going well in Italy—amazingly so. While the rate of obesity in Mississippi is 37 percent, in northern Italy it seems to be stuck at just under 8 percent. Both regions suffered brutal pellagra epidemics. A century later, one is unusually skinny and the other is unusually fat.

The reason seems obvious enough. Southerners gorge on fried chicken, smothered pork chops, and barbecue and wash it all down with sweet tea, while Italians dine on grilled fish and roast vegetables kissed with droplets of extra-virgin olive oil.

That stereotype is nowhere close to being true. Olive oil may seem the embodiment of Italian cuisine, but northern Italians, unlike southerners, also love butter. The average American consumes about thirty-five pounds of cheese per year, which is generally regarded as a grave contributor to the obesity epidemic, but northern Italians outperform Americans by several pounds. Since Roman times, the region has enjoyed a delicacy called *lardo*, which consists of pork fat cured it in salt and herbs. *Lardo* can be cut into thin strips that melt on your mouth, or it can be whipped it into a kind of buttery spread.

If a single location epitomizes the region's love of fat, it is the city of Bologna, the birthplace of the notoriously fatty luncheon meat. Locals call it mortadella, and unlike American bologna, this version is flecked with little cubes of white fat. The city of Bologna has its own version of the veal cutlet, which takes the standard breaded and fried cutlet and drapes it in ham and melted cheese. In Bologna, it is not unusual to go out for a *gran fritto misto*, a meal in which every single course, including dessert, is fried—fried lamb, fried chicken, fried mortadella, fried sweetbreads, fried mozzarella cheese balls, fried zucchini, and fried custard. But Bologna's most influential contribution to world cuisine—more famous, even, than bologna—is *ragù alla bolognese*, the classic Italian meat sauce. Despite what many non-Italians may believe, it does not contain any garlic or tomatoes or bundles of fresh vegetables and herbs. Its main ingredients are pancetta (cured pork belly), ground beef, beef stock, a squirt of tomato paste, and full-fat milk.

All that fat is a mere accompaniment to another controversial and apparently deadly macronutrient: carbs. Refined, high-glycemic, calorie-rich carbohydrates. Northern Italians love them. Take white rice as an example. Italians generally do not eat it much, except for northerners, who are fond of a dish called risotto, which is usually cooked with butter, broth, and grated cheese and stirred until creamy. Northern Italians also adore polenta, particularly in the Veneto region, as well as bread, which comes in numerous superb varieties. Nor are they strangers to sugar. The region's formidable contribution to the world of sweets includes tiramisu, panettone, zabaglione, panna cotta, and gelato. The otherwise unknown town called Longarone bills itself the City of Gelato.

No examination of Italian cuisine, of course, may be had without a discussion of pasta. In Bologna, one noodle in particular, the tagliatella, which is made from eggs and flour looks like fettuccine, is prized above all others. To say this city worships tagliatelle is in no way an exaggeration. The chamber of commerce houses a golden tagliatella, which, like the International Prototype of the Kilogram, represents the official, perfect standard—exactly eight millimeters wide and just over a millimeter thick. A group calling itself Gli Apostoli della Tagliatella—the Apostles of the Tagliatella—holds meetings at restaurants and generally endeavors to preserve the tradition of what they consider the queen of pastas.

The king of pastas is not a noodle. It is a dumpling, the tortellino, a small ring of dough stuffed with a blend of roasted pork loin, mortadella, Parmesan cheese, prosciutto, eggs, and nutmeg. The tortellino, like tagliatelle, has inspired its own sect, called the Learned Brotherhood of the Tortellino. Its senior members wear flowing golden robes made of cotton and silk, and the president wears a medallion. According to the brotherhood, there is one true way to serve tortellini: floating in a broth made from beef and a farmyard chicken.

The official recipe for tortellini is registered at the chamber of commerce, as is the recipe for *ragù alla bolognese*. As are the recipes for the *gran fritto misto alla bolognese*, the lasagna, the fried cheese and mortadella sticks, the mortadella mousse, the veal cutlet with ham and melted cheese, and a dish consisting of sausage wrapped in beef.

CONSIDER ALL of this for a moment. This is a city that gave its name to a fatty deli meat, where entire meals are fried and grown men and women express a religious devotion to pasta, and whose Chamber of Commerce keeps a noodle cast in gold. It is situated, furthermore, in a chunk of geography known for its love of rice and polenta. According to everything we have been taught about the weight-adding effects of fat and carbs and how blends of salt, sugar, and fat are beyond our ability to resist, Bologna should be the Jackson, Mississippi, of Italy.

The scientists who study obesity these days tend to regard the condition in evolutionary terms. Humans, the thinking goes, developed in an environment where calories were hard to come by, and an individual who was inclined to store them as fat had an advantage over someone who was not. This is called the thrifty gene hypothesis, but it's easier to think of it as the Hungry Ape Theory of obesity: our primitive, animalistic brains are wired to be hungry, permanently preparing for famine. Just as you can't be too rich, you can't have too many stored calories.

This strategy, the thinking goes, worked twenty thousand years ago, when a single good meal was hard to come by. Fast-forward to the present, and this same calorie-obsessed, Stone Age brain has been plunked into what scientists refer to as "the modern food environment," where calories are cheap and calories are everywhere. You can't walk a hundred yards in a mall without your brain being tempted by Cinnabon, pizza, cheeseburgers, or caramel popcorn. Engineered for maximum calorie consumption, our brains take in food the way a sponge soaks up water.

By that reckoning, Italy ought to be the most deadly food environment in the world. Its food is so exceptionally good that it attracts nearly one foreign tourist for every resident. (That is four times the US rate.) When the World Food Travel Association, a nonprofit based in Portland, Oregon, conducted a survey asking nearly three thousand travelers from eleven different countries to rate the destination with the "best food, beverage or culinary experiences for travelers," 80 percent of respondents chose Italy—more than any other country. A country with just 0.8 percent of the world's population is the fifth most visited country on the planet.

So for everyone who thinks delicious food is what makes people fat, here are some blunt statistics. The average Italian man—a hungry male ape living in the world's most delicious food environment—weighs 170 pounds. The average American man, by comparison, weighs 200 pounds. Between 1980 and 2008, the average American woman gained around 20 pounds—the most among women in any high-income country. In that same period, according to a study published in the *Lancet*, Italian women seem to have *lost* weight. In the decade that followed, the number of obese Italian eight- and nine-year-olds decreased by thirty thousand.

In America today, 70 percent of women are either overweight or obese. In northern Italy, it is the inverse: 70 percent of women are thin. And of the remaining 30 percent, the vast majority are merely overweight. If you put 1,000 random American women in a room, 115 of them would have "severe obesity"—a five-foot-four-inch woman, for example, weighing 237 pounds. In Italy, there would be three such women. What could possibly explain this?

There are theories. For example, perhaps Italians have perfected the practice of self-discipline. This is possible, but highly

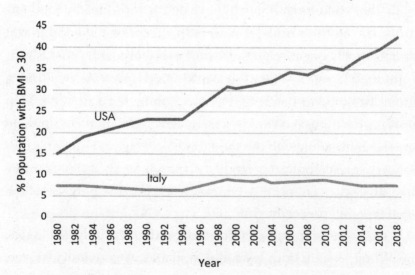

Historic Rates of Obesity in the USA and Italy

improbable. For one thing, given that Italian food is tastier than American food, Italians would need to exert even more self-discipline to resist it. Frankly, they don't seem up to it. Besides the Apostles of the Tagliatella and the Learned Brotherhood of the Tortellino, Bologna is also home to Lamborghini and Maserati as well as the world's largest ice-cream-machine company. Self-restraint does not seem to be in the city's DNA.

Some believe that Italians are trim because they eat a "traditional" diet, that they never gave up the old ways. Also wrong. The change in Italian eating over the last century is at least as dramatic as the change in American eating. Since the 1950s olive oil and vegetable consumption are down. Italian men have doubled the amount of meat they eat and more than doubled cheese consumption, while Italian women have tripled the amount of meat they eat and more than quadrupled servings of dessert. Their cheese intake is nearly *five times* what it used to be. It seems like a recipe for weight gain—more meat, more cheese, more dessert. But it isn't, because Italians' intake has dwindled by more than half. And if that sounds like an endorsement of low-carb eating, it isn't. Italians barely had obesity fifty years ago when they consumed a tremendously carb-rich diet, and they barely have it now.

Biology is another possible explanation. Perhaps Italians are the owners of the much-coveted "thin gene." While theoretically possible, this, too, is false. Given the right circumstances, Italians are as capable as anyone at gaining weight. When Italians migrate to America, Australia, or even to Switzerland, they put on weight. Outside Italy, in fact, being Italian looks more like a disadvantage when it comes to weight gain.

It isn't due to a lack of junk food, either. In Italy, Big Macs and Whoppers are both legal and available, as is Kentucky Fried

Chicken by the bucket. Potato chips come in distinctive Italian flavors, such as porchetta, carbonara, and pesto. The average Italian drinks a third as much of soft drink as the average American, but should the urge arise, little fridges at convenience stores all over the country are well stocked with Coke, Nestea, and Fanta.

Which brings us to the Mediterranean diet. This famous way of eating, discovered by the legendary physiologist Ancel Keys in the late 1950s, was popularized by stories of cultures in southern Europe living longer and having less disease because they eat a diet rich in whole grains, fish, legumes, and vegetables. It has long been assumed that the Mediterranean diet explains Italy's, and particularly northern Italy's, striking thinness. Unfortunately, it overlooks a critical point: while southern Italians do consume more olive oil, more fish, and less meat, they not only weigh more than northern Italians, they also suffer from more heart disease. If Ancel Keys were alive today, he would find that the thinnest women in Italy aren't eating legumes, fish, and whole grains. They are well educated northern Italian divorcées who smoke and consume six or more alcoholic drinks per week.

The truth is, no one can explain why northern Italians are so thin, not even the experts. This is forgivable. What is less forgivable is that so many of the scientists who study obesity don't seem to be aware of northern Italians' trimness. If you corner one of them at a meeting and mention the 8 percent figure, they seem caught by surprise. After a moment of awkward silence, they assure you there is nothing special at all about northern Italy, that whatever advantage it may appear to have is just an illusion, and one that won't last. "Italy," one scientist, who seemed almost annoyed that I could have asked something so naive, told me over the phone, "is just twenty years behind us, that's all."

Is that so? Because twenty years ago the national rate of obesity in the United States was 33.7 percent. In Italy today it is 8.9 percent or 7.6 percent, depending on what statistics you consult. No one can even say the last time America was that thin, because in 1960, when the Centers for Disease Control began keeping track, obesity already stood at 13.4 percent. If Italy is "behind" the United States, it is behind by more than sixty years.

Except Italy isn't "behind." Something is keeping Italians thin. It isn't genes, it isn't self-discipline, it isn't junk food, and it isn't the Mediterranean diet. What is their secret?

If you look back far enough into each country's history, a significant difference emerges that might be a clue. Each country was on a similar nutritional path when a fork appeared in the road. What caused the split? The way each country eliminated pellagra. So the question must be asked, Could the use of vitamins have something to do with it? Is it possible that tinkering with the basic nature of food led to some unintended consequence that would rear its ugly head decades later?

As nutritional theories go, this one is painful to contemplate. To even consider that vitamins—nature's sacred promoters of wellness and vitality—could play a role in obesity seems staggeringly foolish. Vitamins contain no dietary energy or calories. As their name suggests, they are *vital* to the most basic functioning of living organisms. You can't live without them, as pellagra so vividly demonstrated. How could they be bad?

Then again, how is it that the citizens of Bologna are skinny? Maybe carbs and fat and sugar are not always the evil agents we suspect them to be. Perhaps the truth about eating and body weight is not what we think, because when it comes to food, we do not understand *how* we think.

PART II

You Are a Metabolic Genius

(and You Love It)

3

You're Hot. Then You're Not

You are hot. Your forehead is dappled with sweat, you are thirsty, and you feel light-headed. A bucket of cold water is in front of you. You plunge your hand in. How does it feel?

(a) unpleasant
(b) pleasant

In 1963 the official answer was (a) unpleasant. Water felt best at 91°F, as proven by scientific tests. The pleasantness or unpleasantness of water had to do with skin. The further away its temperature moved from 91°F, the more unpleasant a person felt. If a howling winter lowered skin temperature, you *felt* cold. If the steamy air of a torrid sauna raised skin temperature, you *felt* hot. It was straightforward and simple. It was in all the textbooks.

Then Michel Cabanac rinsed the bathtub.

A physiologist at the University of Lyon, Cabanac had just completed an experiment that required him to sit in a tub of hot water until his internal core temperature had risen above normal. His forehead was dappled with sweat, he felt thirsty and light-headed, and the subject for the next experiment was due to arrive at any moment. Still too junior to afford an assistant, Cabanac had to scrub down the tub with bleach between tests, which only made him hotter. As he began the final rinse, Cabanac turned on the cold tap and let the water flow over his hand. It was cold and bracing. And it felt wonderful. According to the textbooks, this was not possible. What was going on?

There and then, Cabanac decided to perform an experiment on his next subject. When he arrived, Cabanac inserted a temperature probe in the man's mouth and another in his rectum, filled the freshly scrubbed bathtub with hot water, and asked the man to get in. In time, the thermometers indicated that the man's core temperature had risen above normal, at which point Cabanac placed a tank of very cold water next to the tub and asked the man to put his hand in it.

"How does it feel?"

"Very pleasant," the man reported.

Next, Cabanac dumped ice in the bath. The water cooled, and slowly the man's core temperature drifted down to normal, eventually dipping below. Cabanac did the tank test again, but now the results were reversed. The cold water that had felt soothing just minutes ago now felt unpleasant. A tank of warm water, on the other hand, now felt wonderful.

The pleasantness of cold water, Cabanac realized in a bolt of insight, wasn't determined by the temperature of that water, or even the temperature of a person's skin: it depended on the body. Somewhere deep inside the human sanctum, there must be a temperature sensor, a tiny thermometer bobbing in the river of blood. When it registered a problematic rise in temperature, coldness felt good. A decline, on the other hand, made warmth feel good. The water temperature that felt best came down to which one returned the body to its preferred internal state. If conditions changed in the environment—if a hot bath became cold—the brain changed plans accordingly. Human beings, Cabanac realized, are career temperature regulators. We open windows, turn up the heat, and steal the covers in the middle of night, all in a lifelong effort to keep the internal temperature just right.

For decades, scientists had missed what Cabanac discovered, and the reason was *because* they were scientists. In their efforts to be "rigorous"—to make sure no aspect of the experiment itself was affecting the results—they had always tested the pleasantness of warm or cold water on people sitting in a lukewarm room. Their brains, therefore, had no reason to reach a temperature equilibrium. In hindsight, it seems like a clumsy oversight. But, as Michel Cabanac says, "Nothing is more difficult to study than the obvious."

Behind our deepest urges and inclinations, Cabanac found, lay a startling intelligence, and he would perform numerous experiments that demonstrated its power. In one study, his test subjects were seated in a frigid room wearing only a bathing suit while a fan blasted cold air at them. In front of them sat a money counter, with a number slowly ticking up. The longer a person could withstand the cold, the more money he or she would take home. Each subject had a breaking point, where the pain of being cold finally overwhelmed the thought of all that money. But it wasn't a fixed point. If Cabanac paid them more money—if the counter ticked up faster—the research subjects lasted longer. In the most literal sense, money could buy pain.

An internal computation was taking place, but it was unconscious. Cabanac's research subjects didn't sit there dispassionately weighing their level of pain against the size of their upcoming rent check. No one had a calculator or an abacus. It was as though somewhere deep in the mind there was a scale, with money on one side and the pain of being cold on the other. As long as the thought of money outweighed its opponent, the subject would sit shivering in agony. But once the sensation of coldness tipped the scale, the subject would flee the room with his winnings.

Not only was this inner system lightning fast, it was deeply in touch with the innermost workings of the body. In another experiment, Cabanac had his subjects walk on a treadmill, but also gave them control of the room's thermostat. As he increased the machine's slope, making it steeper and forcing his subjects to work harder, his human guinea pigs lowered the room temperature because the cool felt soothing. Their chosen reduction in room temperature, Cabanac found, was accurate to an uncanny degree—it was directly proportional to the heat their muscles produced. The simple, impulsive act of turning down the thermostat produced the optimal physiological state.

When it came to body temperature, what felt good was healthy.

A FEW years after the bathtub revelation, Cabanac began thinking about eating. If the body was so good at regulating its temperature, he thought, perhaps it had a similar ability to regulate body weight. This certainly seemed to be the case for Cabanac himself. Until then, he'd never had to think much about how much he weighed. As a child during World War II and the lean years that followed, his favorite food was rutabaga. With postwar prosperity the national food situation improved, and Cabanac grew to love the delicacies of France—Roquefort cheese, lobster à *l'américaine*, blood sausage with sautéed apples, potatoes au gratin. Food brought him considerable pleasure and appeared well tailored to his physiological requirements. He ate as he pleased, and he stayed trim. He was thirty-five years old and weighed 150 pounds, just as he had for most of his adult life.

It did not work that way for everyone, however. Some people clearly ate much more food than they "needed," and it was generally assumed to be a fault of character—their fatness was nothing more than the consequence of a long history of self-indulgence. To Cabanac, this made no sense. If urges were related to the "needs of the body," why would anyone feel the urge to eat more than was required?

It was time for more experiments. In one of them, Cabanac asked his superior, a respected physiologist named Joseph Chatonnet, to fast for twelve hours. The next morning, Cabanac fed him toffees. The first tasted superb to the ravenous Chatonnet. So did the second. After a number of candies, however, the deliciousness began to fade. Now the toffees were just good, and soon they were neither good nor bad. Eventually, to Chatonnet's surprise, he couldn't stand them anymore. In the space of a single morning, toffees went from wonderful to awful.

Perhaps the problem, Cabanac thought, was that the taste of toffee simply became boring after a while. He tested that theory by repeating the experiment with sugar water. When people were hungry, the sugar water tasted good. As they drank more and more, however, each subsequent glass became less alluring, until eventually, as with toffee, sugar water didn't taste good anymore. But there was an important caveat: people had to actually *swallow* the sugar water for its deliciousness to dissipate. If they sipped the sugar water but then spat it out, its deliciousness would persist.

Somewhere deep inside the body, it seemed, a signal was being sent. Just as with temperature, urges were being dictated by the body's internal state—the situation *inside*.

Awed by this metabolic intelligence, Cabanac now conducted his grandest experiment yet: he and two colleagues, American PhD student Herbert Spector and a medical student, Roland Duclaux, set out to lose a great deal of weight. Cabanac aimed to drop twelve pounds—8 percent of his body weight. His two colleagues, who weren't quite as lean, intended to lose 10 percent.

On the first day, before anyone had lost so much as an ounce, the three men established a baseline. Each took a small sip of some sugar water, then took a bottle of orange syrup, removed the cap, and sniffed its aroma. When they were hungry, the sugar water tasted good and the aroma of the orange syrup was captivating. The three men then each drank a glass of water with twelve teaspoons of sugar stirred in—about two hundred calories. An hour later, they repeated the test, sipping sugar water and taking a whiff of the orange syrup. The allure, they found, had vanished. When offered sweet calories, it seemed the brain was saying, "No thank you, I have had enough."

The weight loss began. Cabanac, who normally consumed seventeen hundred calories per day, went down to less than five hundred—the equivalent of a glass of apple juice and three slices of bread with butter. Like millions of people who have played the dieting game, he became obsessed with precisely how much food he consumed. He would bring his little kitchen scale with him everywhere he went, scribbling calculations to figure out what was okay to eat and how much. Losing weight, he discovered, was unexpectedly easy. The pounds practically fell off.

Then weight loss came to an abrupt halt. Cabanac found himself trapped in a valley from which he could not escape. His caloric intake had nose-dived, but the reading on the scale wouldn't budge. Every waking moment was a wrestling match with hunger. At night he would dream of "gorging on mountains of food," only to wake up stricken with guilt, thinking he had ruined the experiment he had worked so hard to produce. He began taking his watch off at weigh-ins—anything to save a few ounces. When he stood on the scale, he felt inclined to inch his feet over to the sides to make the reading lighter. But at last, on the eleventh of December 1970, he reached his target: 138 pounds.

The now lean Cabanac and his two lean colleagues performed the sugar water and orange syrup tests again. On an empty stomach, the sugar water tasted good and the orange syrup smelled wonderful—just as before. But unlike before, gulping down two hundred calories of sugar water did nothing to curb the desire for more calories—the sugar water and orange syrup remained as enticing as ever. Just weeks ago, two hundred calories extinguished Cabanac's hunger. Now the same number of calories seemed to have no effect.

The three men celebrated the end of their experiment with a grand meal at a local restaurant called l'Auberge Savoyarde, which specialized in lyonnaise cuisine. Cabanac effortlessly put away 4,550 calories, tripling in a single meal what he normally downed in a typical day. (One of his colleagues consumed 7,945 calories.) In the weeks that followed, Cabanac ate whatever he wanted whenever he wanted, with no restrictions. He gained weight effortlessly and happily and by the middle of March was back at 150 pounds. Then, without any effort on Cabanac's part, the weight gain came to a halt. He continued to eat as he pleased, to indulge in the French foods he so loved, but he remained, almost as though he were stuck, at 150 pounds.

He was back in his old familiar body. Cabanac performed the sugar water and orange syrup tests a last time. Gulping down two hundred calories once again turned off his appetite. His inner calorie counter said, "Enough." Humans, Cabanac now realized, were not universally programmed to ravenously overeat. Body weight, like temperature, seemed to have a preferred setting, which he referred to as a "set point." For years, Cabanac's weight never rose above his set point, which was at 150 pounds. But when it fell below that level, visions of food seized control of Cabanac's mind, and when he ate, it took more food to make him feel full.

His body was behaving just like that of a person whose core temperature had slipped a degree. The urge for food was guiding Cabanac back to the optimal internal state. There was an inner program and it knew exactly what it was doing.

It seems obvious when you step back. Food calls out to you when you're hungry. People don't feel like eating when they're full. Nothing, however, is more slippery than the obvious. Most of us carry on as though the appetite is dangerously out of control, or that if there is such a thing as a set point, it's at 450 pounds. We try to battle our inner programming by eating less, eating more vegetables, or burning off all those calories with exercise. We have taken every possible strategy to bring our frenzied urges under control. What is dieting, after all, but the official recognition that the body's natural inclinations must be regulated.

It always works. In the early stages, dieting consistently delivers results, often spectacularly. The stories you see on TV of people "miraculously" losing ten pounds in a single week are true. Every diet works. I repeat: every diet works. Just not for long.

As the body begins burning more calories than it's taking in, it starts to raid its inner reserve of carbohydrates, called glycogen, which is stored in water in the muscles and the liver. Water is heavy, and as all that water disappears, the pounds appear to melt away. Jeans that were too tight become flatteringly snug. People stop you on the street and tell you how great you look. It can happen in as little as a few days. The miracle, however, soon gives way to something akin to trench warfare. As Michel Cabanac discovered firsthand, you can spend a week fighting an exhausting battle over a few ounces that ends in stalemate. Around the six- to eight-month mark, weight loss hits a plateau. People exercise. They forgo dessert. They swear they are still eating less, but the pounds begin to come back, as if the body were manufacturing flesh out of thin air. People snap back to set point. The internal program has made its decision about body weight. Good luck fighting it.

As surprising as this may sound, the inflexibility of the human brain about body weight has been known for at least a half century. In 1959, a physician named Jules Hirsch discovered first-hand the stubborn nature of obesity. Four of his patients, who collectively weighed 1,290 pounds, lived at Rockefeller University Hospital for eight months and subsisted for months on a liquid diet that delivered six hundred calories per day, a fraction of their requirement. It appeared to be a smashing success. Each patient lost an average of a hundred pounds, and the day they were discharged, everyone, including Jules Hirsch, welcomed the new, thinner, happier life that awaited them. But they quickly gained it all back. They sprang back to their old weight, just like Michel

Cabanac. The months spent living in a hospital on a meager liquid diet were all wasted.

Hirsch did more experiments. When obese people lost weight, he found, they underwent profound physiological changes. Their heart rate dropped, they became sensitive to cold temperatures, and their white blood cell count dwindled. It was a total mind-body ordeal. They became anxious and depressed and had suicidal thoughts. Time seemed to slow to a crawl. His subjects would hide food in their rooms and become embarrassed and remorseful when they got caught. They would have vivid dreams of eating. Even the way they perceived their own bodies became distorted. When they would look at photographs of their now-thin selves, they opted to "correct" the image by looking at it with a distorting lens that returned their bodies to their former larger state.

The results were uncannily similar to those of people who were starving—specifically, a group of conscientious objectors to World War II who were intentionally deprived of food to study starvation's effects. Those subjects lost interest in everything, including sex, and became obsessed with food. One man secretly ate several sundaes and malted milks and stole candy. Another ate scraps of food pulled out of garbage cans. Another chewed forty packs of gum per day. Another man, passing a bakery, bought a dozen doughnuts and handed them out to children, just for the joy of watching them eat. "If you went to a movie," one subject reminisced, years later, "you weren't particularly interested in the love scenes, but you noticed every time they ate and what they ate."

Peak pain was experienced during "refeeding," when hunger could not be satisfied no matter how much food the men ate. The amounts consumed were staggering: one of the subjects put away six thousand calories in a single meal and was back snacking an hour later. Another had to have his stomach pumped.

It was the same with Hirsch's patients. "To all appearances," he wrote, "our weight-reduced patients were experiencing starvation." The technical term is *semistarvation neurosis*. Only they weren't starving.

The brain is not some bumbling, famished imbecile trapped in that warm liquid attic, perpetually barking out orders to eat. The brain regulates body mass as keenly as it regulates temperature. Fat cells release hormones that tell the brain how much fat there is. Scientists recently discovered sensors in leg bones of rodents that seem to track body weight. Adolescent girls begin to develop sexually not when they reach a certain age, but when they reach a certain *weight*. The brain, on some level, "knows" precisely how heavy the body is. Roughly above your throat sits a pea-size piece of gray matter where cells that crank up the drive to eat have been found. When people go on diets, these cells turn on—not a big surprise. These cells are *turned off*, similarly, by the hormone released by fat cells.

You would never know this by watching what a person eats. Food intake is like a yo-yo, up one day, down the next. During any given day, the amount a person eats is almost never the same as the amount that person expends. How could it be? We eat in concentrated little bursts but expend energy constantly. As you sit there munching, you consume energy at a rate five times higher than you burn it during intense exercise.

In April 1981, scientists began tracking for one year the day-to-day "customary" eating of twenty-nine typical Americans going about life as normal. One woman's daily food diaries revealed spikes of eye-popping overconsumption. She ate 3,140 calories one day in mid-August. Two days later, she consumed 3,718 calories—an intake appropriate to a three-hundred-pound man. The holidays were a swamp of indulgence—2,395 calories one day, 2,623 the day after. Then, three days after that, she capped the magnificent week of feasting with a yearly high of 3,788 calories.

How much weight had this 145-pound woman gained one year later? None. There were high-calorie days, certainly. But there were also lean days—and more of the latter than the former. Over the weeks and months, she somehow achieved *balance*. And she achieved it exactly. She ended the year a titch over 146 pounds, which is, as the scientists say, statistically insignificant. It was as though behind the scenes some master accountant was bringing credits and debits into alignment.

That master accountant is astoundingly precise. Kevin Hall— the scientist whose study showed that carbs perform similarly to fat when it comes to weight loss—performed an experiment that crisply illustrates the appetite's astonishing gift for precision. It followed 153 subjects taking the drug canagliflozin, which diverts sugar from the bloodstream into the urine. Every day, these people were unknowingly peeing away 360 calories worth of sugar. The weight loss should have been spectacular. All of those diverted calories should have added up to a loss of more than twenty-five pounds over a year. But that is not what happened. The brain registered something was amiss, and those oblivious pill-takers unconsciously began eating more food. Every lost pound was matched by a surge in appetite until each subject was obliviously consuming an extra 350 calories per day—almost exactly the same number of calories they were losing in their urine.

Not only are the body's urges precise, they are stubborn, tenacious, and unwavering. In 2009, Kevin Hall began studying the contestants competing on *The Biggest Loser*, the reality show on which very large people compete to see who can lose the most weight. After thirty weeks of vigorous exercise and diet, the show served up truly Hollywood-level results, with the average weight dropping from 328 to 202 pounds. Collectively, the competitors removed more than fifteen hundred pounds of fat from their frames. Their bodies weren't just slimmer, however. They ran differently. Their "resting metabolic rate," which refers to the energy required just to stay running—to breathe, pump blood, blink, and yawn—had slowed down. Some of this was expected, because it takes less energy to run a smaller body, the same way it takes less gas to power a smaller car. But the drop was too big. On average, each contestant was using 275 *fewer* calories per day than expected—about half a Big Mac's worth—just to function. They were running in super-economy mode.

Six years later, Hall performed a follow-up study that assessed the progress of fourteen of the original sixteen contestants. Some of the news was good. On average, they all gained back ninety pounds, which may sound bad but is much less than one would expect. One of the contestants did spectacularly well, losing an additional thirty-one pounds.

In other ways, though, the picture was deflating. Every other contestant gained weight. Three had bounced back to their initial weight, one was twenty-nine pounds heavier, and one was a full fifty-four pounds heavier than the day the contest began. It sounds like a classic failure of willpower—those gluttonous and lazy "regainers" strayed back to their old indulgent ways. But that's not what happened at all. The contestants were still exercising. They were still eating less. On average, each was now consuming 375 fewer calories per day than when the competition had started. By all rights, they should have been skinnier.

The problem was that their bodies had changed. They were experiencing "persistent metabolic adaptation." Their metabolisms were stuck in economy mode. They were now burning a full 499 fewer calories per day than expected—almost an entire Big Mac's worth. No matter how hard they tried, they were losing the war on calories. Six years on, it was as though the contest never actually ended.

AND NOW for the most surprising fact of all: The brain doesn't just resist losing weight. It resists *gaining* weight. Really and truly. When weight dips below a certain point, the brain goes into starvation mode and fights like hell to get it back up. But if it rises above set point, the brain also fights—like hell, in some cases—to bring the weight back down. It goes against our most deep-seated beliefs about our fraught relationship to food—that fatness is the body's true aim.

The first person to take note of this was a German scientist named Rudolf Otto Neumann, who, in 1902, while experimenting on himself, noticed his weight remained oddly stable whether he ate a lot or a little. It was as if the body had some way of getting rid of unwanted energy—an overflow valve for unneeded calories.

Decades later, Ethan Sims, a scientist at the University of Vermont, witnessed a similar phenomenon when he attempted to fatten his lab mice. He provided them with all the tasty food they could eat, but, despite his efforts, the mice stayed trim. If he force-fed them, the mice would compensate by burning extra calories and gain less than expected. And as soon as the force-feeding was stopped, skinniness returned.

Frustrated by rodents, Sims turned to students. Hungry college students, he believed, would get fat if given enough food. They, too, however, remained stubbornly trim. So, like Joseph Goldberger so many years before, Sims moved on to inmates at a local state prison. This time his fattening experiment worked, but Sims discovered it was anything but easy to get the inmates to gain weight. With time, the very thought of food came to disgust them, and participants began to drop out of the study. Those that remained spent months eating as much as ten thousand calories per day, but their weight only increased by around 25 percent. The gain seemed too small. Just as dieters conserve calories at all costs, the overstuffed prisoners began expending them.

Some of this is expected—larger bodies require more calories to move and to keep running than smaller ones. But the increase was too large. Just to stay obese, Sims observed, his subjects had to eat more food than a "naturally" obese person of the same weight. Then, when the experiment was over, all but one of the subjects dropped back to his initial body weight.

More than thirty years after Jules Hirsch witnessed his patients bounce back to their original weights, an older and wiser Jules Hirsch undertook one of the more unusual experiments in the history of physiology. Obese as well as non-obese test subjects were overfed or underfed. When body weight was reduced by 10 percent, everyone's metabolism tightened up—the obese and non-obese alike. But astonishingly, when body weight was raised by 10 percent, everyone—the obese included—burned extra calories. Metabolic adaptation is a two-way street. Even for people with obesity. There wasn't some fundamental biological difference between the obese and the thin. People with obesity are not beset by an insatiable greed for food. The difference came down to their internal target. They gravitated to different weights and fought hard to stay there.

If this all seems too hard to believe, just ask the Masa people of northern Cameroon and Chad, who consider fatness to be a sign of wealth and virility among young men. Every year, a small number embark on a period of incredible food intake called the *guru walla*. The aim is to achieve a bulging stomach, large buttocks, and a smooth layer of buttery fat spread over their entire frame. To achieve this, they live in a hut by themselves, often naked, for two months, eating every two hours, give or take, from six in the morning until four the next morning. They can leave the hut only to milk cows or defecate, which can take place up to five times a day. A typical day goes as follows: porridge, porridge, porridge, sorghum paste, milk, porridge, porridge, sorghum loaf and relish, porridge, porridge, milk.

The level of food intake is spectacular. In 1976, a *guru walla* participant ate more than seventeen pounds of food in a single day, totaling 16,823 calories—the caloric equivalent of a wheelbarrow filled with thirty Big Macs. By the end of his *guru walla*, he'd gained sixty-four pounds. A fellow participant who gained seventy-five pounds couldn't get up without using a stick for help.

"The feeding hours," two French anthropologists described, "are punctuated by a good deal of vomiting, farting, defecating, and urinating." It is a battle. The Masa men have to sit upright, with their heads held just so to keep themselves from vomiting out the food they've worked so hard to get down.

Here, alas, is the starkest irony of them all. Like the hundreds of millions of frustrated, depressed dieters on the other side of the

planet—the millions who lose weight only to find it comes back—
the Masa cannot maintain their ideal, hard-won weight. Over the
months that follow, that fabulous buttery sheen disappears, and—
snap!—they are back where they started. They want to be fat. But
they are doomed to be thin.

4

The Quest for Pleasure

The brain—clearly, obviously, undeniably—is a metabolic genius. If you assembled the world's greatest minds and provided each with the world's fastest supercomputer, they, collectively, could not keep a running tally of our biological needs, let alone keep them perpetually in check. The brain does it effortlessly. Twenty-four hours a day, every day of every week.

The big fatty blob of neurons that controls breathing, heart rate, and blinking is the very same big fatty blob of neurons that fills out tax returns and brews coffee. These two departments, however, are sealed off from each other. No matter how hard we concentrate, we can't raise or lower our body temperature any more than we can mentally control how much we weigh. We all act as though we are the unquestioned captains of our own ship. But the truth is that we have little say in so much of what we think and do.

And so, a question: If the brain senses change in the body and computes that action is required, how does it achieve its intended result? It is one thing to realize food is needed, but quite another to procure a meal and consume it. How does the brain translate all that information and computation into action?

* * *

EVEN IF you have never heard the name Howard Moskowitz, there is a good chance you have experienced his work. Moskowitz is a psychophysicist who spent a remarkable career discovering the unusual but often fantastic quirks of human taste, such as that a portion of society prefers orange juice with lots of pulp. He is best known for his discovery that some people like their tomato sauce chunky, which Malcolm Gladwell wrote about in his book *What the Dog Saw*. Moskowitz is also famous for the creation of Cherry Vanilla Dr Pepper, which he engineered by tinkering with combinations of flavorings and sugar until his concoction tickled the now famous "bliss point," as the investigative journalist Michael Moss described in his book *Salt Sugar Fat*.

But if you ask Moskowitz, he will tell you all that work pales in comparison to his life's greatest discovery. It sits, buried and long forgotten, in the December 1975 issue of *Science*—one of the world's most prestigious scientific journals—in a crisp two-pager called "Cross-Cultural Differences in Simple Taste Preferences."

The article described two experiments that were conducted at St. John's Medical College in Bangalore, India. In the first, a group of Indian medical students tasted several samples of sugar water, each one sweeter than the last, and rated them for pleasantness. They then did the same thing with sour water. The thinking was that sweet was pleasant and sour was unpleasant, and that this was a hardwired response that was the same for all humans. It's how we come out of the womb.

Lo and behold, it is how Indian medical students come out of the womb. Like humans everywhere, they didn't like sour, but sweet was good and got better and better until it reached the glorious bliss point. (Beyond the bliss point, sugar water tastes too sweet.)

Next up was a group of laborers from the outlying region of Karnataka, the state of which Bangalore is the capital. These men were poor, and most of them could not read or write. But they had a trait that caught Moskowitz's attention: a predilection for eating extremely sour food, particularly tamarind, a local tropical pod fruit that hangs from trees. Some tamarind is sweet, such as the variety grown in Thailand, which can contain as much as 48 percent sugar. The variety grown in Karnataka, which is less sweet, can contain as little as 5 percent. Unripe tamarind is both the sourest and the cheapest, and therefore more affordable for poor laborers. They would use it dishes such as roti or lentil stew. Sometimes, they chewed it raw.

Moskowitz was curious if these people's experience of sourness followed the standard model. Since his test subjects couldn't read or write, Moskowitz had to devise some way for them to convey their opinions of each liquid. His solution was to have them draw little vertical bars. The more delicious the liquid, the more bars they were instructed to draw.

It all went as expected with the sugar water. More sweetness generated more bars until, at last, the bliss point was reached. When it came to sweetness, their preferences matched the established human standard. With the sour test, however, things got interesting. As the samples got progressively sourer, the more lines appeared on the score sheets. These people *liked* sour. The liking curve, as Moskowitz puts it, looked just like the liking curve for sweet. For them, and only them, sour surged to a climactic bliss point of its very own. Here in the middle of southern India was a group of people who loved a taste that humans were not supposed to love. "This sense we thought was built-in to be unpleasant," Moskowitz says, "was showing the behavior of something that was pleasant." The poor, illiterate laborers from Karnataka lived in a different food world.

Karnataka does seem like another world. The place is downright hostile to human life, even though people have been living there for five thousand years. The interior plateau is dry, and the summer temperatures are blazing. One of the few crops that can be grown is called jowar, a relative of corn, which locals bake into the flatbread called roti. As with corn, if people eat too much jowar and not enough of anything else, they get pellagra. Since jowar is the number one crop in Karnataka, the disease has been known to sweep through the region in spring, just it would do in northern Italy and the American South.

It's a good thing, then, that the laborers ate all that tamarind. This peculiar sour fruit contains nearly three times as much niacin, by weight, than milk—quite a lot for a fruit or vegetable. As hostile to living as Karnataka might be, it does come with an unexpected bonus: the remedy to pellagra grows on trees.

Pellagra, however, is the least of Karnataka's nutritional troubles. A much larger problem is the water supply, which is overloaded with fluoride. Most people recognize this element for its role in preventing cavities. It forms a chemical bond with tooth enamel, which makes teeth harder and less susceptible to decay. But if a person consumes too much fluoride, it disrupts the body's mineral metabolism, causing a toxic condition called fluorosis. In milder cases, a person's teeth will become stained and pitted. In severe cases, excess fluoride disturbs the formation of bone, resulting in horribly deformed limbs, fractures that won't heal, and hideous cases of hunchback. It rains so rarely in Karnataka that villagers pump water from deep underground, where it has long been marinating in fluoride. They drink it, they cook with it, and slowly they become poisoned. If that weren't bad enough, eating jowar exacerbates fluoride's toxic effects. When it comes to fluorosis, Karnataka is a perfect storm.

Luckily, it also has the perfect solution.

Twenty-four years after Moskowitz's groundbreaking findings, a scientist at India's National Institute of Nutrition named Arjun Khandare began experimental feedings of fluoride and tamarind to dogs. It had long been known that tamarind gel possessed a "fluoride entrapment capacity"—if you added it to water, it could remove 80 percent of the element. There had been all sorts of attempts to solve the fluorosis problem, but none of them worked. The hope was that tamarind might help.

In the experiment, a group of dogs fed fluoride was compared to dogs fed both fluoride and tamarind. The dogs in the latter group not only excreted more fluoride in their urine, less fluoride accumulated in their bones. Somehow, the tamarind was flushing fluoride out of these dogs' bodies.

The fruit's apparent healing power wasn't some freak phenomenon confined to the laboratory. Around the same time, another Indian scientist set out to solve a rural mystery: cows and bison suffered from fluorosis, but goats and sheep tended not to. This presented a riddle. All four animals are ruminants, and all had access to similar water. In theory, all four species should have been equally susceptible to fluorosis. The difference, the scientist found, came down to what they ate. Sheep and goats are "browsers." Their lips are almost as dexterous as human fingers—they can pluck berries, pods, and leaves off twigs as they eat. Some of these fruits, leaves, and pods that the goats and sheep ate—which included tamarind—contained compounds that protected them from fluoride toxicity. Cows and bison were not so lucky. They are huge beasts that chomp their way through fields of grass—grass that has no antifluoride effects. The healing plants, alas, are unavailable to them, thus making them more predisposed to fluoride's toxic effects.

Following his experiment with dogs, Khandare began testing tamarind on humans. For subjects, he used a group of poverty-stricken boys living in social welfare hostels, where the water they drank was so saturated with fluoride that some were too sick even to be studied. To make matters even worse, one of the hostels had recently started replacing tamarind with tomatoes because they were cheaper. As with the dogs, the boys were fed tamarind and their urine was analyzed. Tamarind, once again, caused a spike in fluoride excretion. It was some kind of super-sour wonder fruit. It even appeared to help remove fluoride that had already been deposited in bone.

Finally, Khandare visited a village where levels of fluoride in its water were so high that roughly half the children had discolored and pitted teeth. The villagers who ate tamarind every day, he found, were healthier than those who ate it only occasionally. Like sheep and goats, they had fewer bone deformities. Their urine not only contained more fluoride, they were half as likely to suffer from a condition called bamboo spine.

AMID ALL these discoveries about tamarind, the most interesting one lay forgotten in a back issue of *Science* from 1975. Moskowitz's discovery of the peculiar sour-loving habits of Karnataka laborers revealed a key insight into human nature. Those laborers knew nothing about fluoride or niacin or the urine-altering power of tamarind. All they knew is this: they liked the way it tastes. The invisible force that drew these people to tamarind wasn't its reputation for "fluoride entrapment capacity," it was the state it induced: bliss. And Moskowitz had made it visible. You could see it on the score sheets—little bars you could count up. Eating tamarind, very simply, felt good.

And that experience—feeling good—is how the brain achieves its goals.

Michel Cabanac called it the quest for pleasure. Humans are on an eternal quest to maximize feeling good and minimize feeling bad. The quest for pleasure is what makes people tolerate the pain of shivering in a cold room, frigid air blasting at them, while they watch a money counter ticking upward. It is what draws the Learned Brothers of the Tortellino to the stuffed little pasta dumpling they so love and moves an Italian city to cast a noodle in gold. The desire to feel good or to avoid pain, as Cabanac puts it, is the "motor that drives that human mind." It is a force as seemingly fundamental as gravity or magnetism—it produces what physicists call "action at a distance." It can make objects move without their being physically touched. Pleasure, simply, is what makes us do things.

In all of Michel Cabanac's experiments, each condition his subjects experienced—hot, cold, money, fatigue—were translated by the brain into the same currency: pleasure. Whether his subjects were shivering in a bathtub of icy water, or whether it was Cabanac himself yearning for food, the mind's impulse was always directed toward what felt good and away from what felt bad. And what felt good was what returned the body's internal state back to its optimal setting. Every impulse we have—to sleep, to sneeze, to peel an orange, pour a glass of wine, get work done, or go to the bathroom—is translated by the brain into a "behavioral final common path." Pleasure is to the mind as money is to the economy. It is the oldest and most fundamental unit of exchange. Maximizing pleasure or minimizing pain, either now or in the future, is how decisions get made. Every decision. Whether you like it or not.

If that strikes you as a radical thought, it was all the more so in Cabanac's day. There was a time in the not-so-distant past when the very idea of "pleasure" was all but laughed at by right-thinking scientists. They weren't clinically depressed or members of an ascetic cult. It was their solemn yet very scientific belief that there was no such thing as pleasure. What people called pleasure or enjoyment or feeling good was a myth, a confused belief about the world that was no more real than the Easter Bunny. These scientists called themselves behaviorists. And as odd as their beliefs may seem today, their mission was governed by a rigorous, if strange, logic.

In the middle of the last century, psychologists tended to come in one of two flavors: behaviorists and Freudians. Freudians were "depth psychologists." They believed in the unconscious, that dreams could be interpreted, and that little boys suffered from an Oedipus complex.

Behaviorists detested Freudians and what they considered to be silly, made-up, and unprovable theories. A psychologist, they believed, should approach the human mind the way a volcanologist approaches a volcano. What a volcanologist does is *measure*—seismic tremors, quantity of ash, gaseous emissions, and so forth. From these data, the volcanologist attempts to make predictions, such as the likelihood the volcano will erupt, or what path the lava flow might take.

The problem with pleasure was that it could not be measured. If a person declared his or her joy over a Philly cheesesteak, you couldn't weigh that feeling or measure its speed or how much space it was taking up. There could never be a roomful of scientists in lab coats all nodding their heads and agreeing that a subject was experiencing 17.34 micrograms of deliciousness. Emotions are, by their nature, private. The only person who "feels good" is the person feeling good—no other person can have access to that feeling. Talking about feelings as though they were real was like saying a volcano was "angry."

So the behaviorists replaced "feelings," which could not be measured, with "drives," which could. Take the phenomenon of thirst as an example. A scientist could measure thirst in a rat by counting the minutes since it last had water, or measuring the concentration of salt in its blood. A scientist could measure the effect of thirst on a rat—how many blocks it would climb to reach its bowl, or how much water it would drink. The concept of "thirst" not only explained both the cause and the effect, it let you *predict* what a rat would do under certain conditions. Thirst, therefore, was nothing more than the "drive" to make the painful state of needing water go away.

That's all the word *pleasure* meant to a behaviorist—a kind of confused term for unpleasantness *going away*. Sex "feels good" because it makes the persistent drive for sex go away. Food "tastes delicious" because it makes hunger, which you can measure and which is another form of pain, go away.

It is called "drive reduction theory" and it ranks among the most cynical and depressing theories of human nature in the history of

science. According to it, there is nothing positive in human existence, just varying shades of negative. Life is an unrelenting cam-
paign to relieve discomfort and make negative "drives" recede.
Feeling good is just feeling less bad. It may seem incomprehensi-
ble, even ridiculous, but at one time this was mainstream science.

All of which makes the events that took place at McGill University, in Montreal, Canada, on a Sunday in 1954 all the more incredible. That afternoon, a Harvard-trained psychologist named
James Olds—a behaviorist—stuck an ultrasharp wire into the
brain of an albino rat and charged it with little zaps of electricity.
Later that evening, he returned home from the lab, greeted his
wife and dropped the following bombshell. He had discovered the
brain's "pleasure center."

Pleasure was real.

Olds was no maverick. His simple experiment was intended
to bolster behaviorism, not destroy it. Olds was aiming his wire
for the part of brain that produced *negative affect*, which was the
technical term for "feeling bad"—the mental state that sat at the
heart of behaviorist theory. Olds thought he had a pretty good idea
where it might be, so he inserted the wire, let the skin heal over,
then placed the rat in an open box. The plan was as follows: The rat,
being curious, would scurry around the box and explore. When
it visited a particular corner, Olds would administer a zap, which
would produce "negative affect" and cause the rat to dread that
particular corner. Olds dubbed this corner of discontent Corner A.

Olds released the rat, the rat visited Corner A, and Olds
zapped it as planned. The rodent, however, did not flee. It didn't
even surreptitiously slink away. It circled and came back to, of all
places, Corner A. Olds zapped it again, as though to correct its
poor judgment, but the animal seemed as content as ever to linger

at Corner A. Whatever brain region that wire had found, it was clearly not the "feeling bad" part.

Olds switched things up. He began zapping the rat's brain when it visited Corner B. Within five minutes, Corner B became the new Corner A. Olds found that he could get the rat to go wherever he wanted by zapping its brain. It was like playing the hot-and-cold game with a child. When it took a step in the right direction, zap. When it got closer, another zap. And when the rat finally got to where Olds wanted it to go, zap zap zap. The rat wanted more. The zaps must have felt good.

In another experiment, Olds starved a rat for twenty-four hours—a very long time for a rat to go without eating—then offered it food. But if he zapped the rat before it got to its meal, the supposedly ravenous rat would just stay put, leaving the food uneaten. To an extremely hungry rat, food is the ultimate reward. Yet one thing topped food: a brain zap.

Next, Olds created levers that the rodents could push themselves. Now they could administer the zaps themselves while Olds stood back and measured "response frequency." The first rat zapped itself. It zapped itself again. It began "self-stimulating" once every five seconds. After thirty minutes, Olds had to turn off the current. The rat just stood there, pressing its lever again and again until it fell asleep.

The appetite for pleasure was insatiable. One rat self-stimulated more than 850,000 times over twenty-one days. When offered the choice between a pleasure lever and food, sleep, sex, or water, the rat would opt for the lever, zapping itself until it collapsed or died. It wasn't just rats. Rabbits, goldfish, pigeons, dogs, cats and chickens all reveled in self-stimulation. A monkey would press its lever three times a second, sixteen hours a day, for *years*. One evening, a dolphin that was inadvertently left in a pool with its wires and switches connected "delighted himself to death after an all-night orgy of pleasure."

Humans were no different. A hungry human, like a hungry rat, preferred pleasure zaps over food. The zaps themselves were said to have something of a sexual quality. Grainy footage from the 1950s shows a chronically depressed woman self-stimulating, her wired cranium covered in a cartoonish wrap of bandage. "I find this button the best," she says. She presses it again and again. "I think it's somewhat of a sexy button."

In one of the strangest and saddest experiments in the history of modern psychology, but one that demonstrates, perhaps more than any other, the power of the brain's pleasure network to guide human behavior, a psychiatrist at Tulane University named Robert Heath attempted to "cure" homosexuality in a disturbed, drug-addicted, tormented young man code named B-19. The doctor placed the patient in a lab along with a twenty-one-year-old prostitute. Thanks to the power of electrical brain stimulation, the study would yield what is undoubtedly one of the strangest sentences in the history of science: "Then, despite the milieu and the encumbrance of the electrode wires, he successfully ejaculated."

- On a December day in 1970, Michel Cabanac effortlessly consumed 4,550 calories at l'Auberge Savoyarde.
- On a September morning in 1976, an eighteen-year-old Masa man in northern Cameroon forced himself to eat two and a half pounds of sorghum porridge and then vomited.

To the external observer, both behaviors appear the same: eating an enormous quantity of food. These two men, however, experienced opposite states. One indulged in unreserved pleasure and the other endured wretched pain.

We think of deliciousness as though it's a fixed attribute. Steak is delicious, so is cherry pie, but cod-liver oil is not. We conceive of deliciousness as though it is as true and universal as temperature or mass. A bowl of ice cream is delicious the way a gallon of water weighs 8.34 pounds.

The harder you look, though, things don't seem to work that way at all. A starving Michel Cabanac craved food so badly he had vivid dreams of eating. But the food he craved isn't what changed—it was Cabanac that had changed. Ethan Sims's overfed prisoners found food so repulsive that some were unable to continue the experiment. But, again, the food they were eating didn't change. It was the prisoners that changed.

The brain is the wizard behind the curtain. It knows how much the body weighs. It knows what it wants the body to weigh. It knows how to get there. And the quest for pleasure is its guide and its fuel.

Michel Cabanac, however, pointed out something we would do well to keep in mind: The body's internal settings are not fixed and unmovable. They can change. They change all the time. Our body temperature of 98.6°F—the universal setting you read about in textbooks—changes every day. Your core is coolest at night and begins warming up just before you wake and reaches its peak again as evening sets in. When challenged by infection, the brain's thermostat resets to a higher temperature. The change in body state is achieved with the universal currency: pleasure. We experience the desire for more warmth. We lie in bed, clutching the duvet and suffering chills until the elevated thermal destination is reached.

The internal settings for body weight and eating can also change. During the long days of summer, the weight of the Siberian hamster seems pinned at forty grams. But if you adjust daylight from sixteen hours to a wintry eight hours, its weight drops up to 40 percent. If you starve the animal during this winter period, it will lose even more weight. If you then give it free rein at the feed dish, it will eat and eat until it reaches its winter set point, but then it will stop. Food seems to instantly loses its allure.

Siberian hamsters, Michel Cabanac, South Indian laborers, and the young Masa men of Africa are all animated by the same invisible force. Pleasure. It is the spark that propels them to eat. And when the pleasure stops, eating stops.

Too Much of a Good Thing

By the 1970s, pleasure had been captured in a bottle. The substance in that bottle was a chemical called dopamine. You have probably heard of it. Dopamine is the "pleasure chemical." Next to insulin, it is one of the few of the body's crucially important chemicals you might hear talked about on TV. It is the fairy dust that causes happiness, elation, and joy.

During the mid-twentieth century, as scientists created an ever more detailed map of the brain, they discovered a highway of dopamine running from the back of the brain right through James Olds's pleasure centers. If you made a dopamine "lesion" in these regions in a rat—killing the dopamine neurons but leaving the others intact—the animal would lose its characteristic sense of curiosity and even stop eating and drinking. Without dopamine, self-stimulation of the brain's pleasure centers would lose its allure until a rat couldn't even be bothered to press its lever. It was also discovered that popular drugs that got people high, such as cocaine and amphetamines, jacked up dopamine levels in the brain. It didn't matter what the source of pleasure—drugs, electrodes, sex, food—if you took dopamine away, pleasure drained away along with it. Dopamine was pleasure, pure and simple. As one scientific paper put it, dopamine was where "sensory inputs are translated into the hedonic messages we experience as pleasure, euphoria or 'yumminess.'"

In 1985, a young neuroscientist named Kent Berridge set out to learn more about this wondrous and crucial brain chemical. He had just spent the past several years studying the facial expressions and gestures rats make when they eat. If a rat liked its food, it would stick its tongue out or lick its paws. If it disliked its food, it would shake its head or open its mouth in a kind of "gape." It had long been thought that this was an automatic reaction—like a reflex. But Berridge helped show these expressions were a true measure of pleasure. If you starved a rat to make it hungry, sugar water would cause a heightened pleasure response. Conversely, if a rat filled up on sugar water, the liquid lost its appeal. It was all controlled by dopamine. Of this, Berridge was "utterly certain."

To add yet more evidence to the theory that dopamine equaled pleasure, Berridge devised a simple experiment. He would administer a dopamine-blocking drug to rats, then squirt sugar water into their mouths to trigger a pleasure response. With the dopamine out of commission, Berridge predicted, the normal response—rats sticking their tongues out or joyously licking their paws—would not occur. The experiment, however, did not turn out as planned. For some unknown reason, the rats gleefully stuck out their tongues, as though the sugar water was as tasty as ever. Berridge presumed he had made some mistake, so he tried it a second time. It happened again. The sugar water remained delicious despite the obstruction of dopamine.

Maybe, Berridge thought, the dopamine blockers just weren't strong enough. So he brought out the heavy artillery: lesions. He chemically destroyed the dopamine pathways in his rats' brains.

The effect was so powerful that the rats were now so totally unin-terested in the delights of eating that they had to be fed through a feeding tube. Once again, Berridge squirted sugar water in their mouths. Without so much as a drop of dopamine left in their brains, there was no way the rats were going to show any signs of enjoyment. But they did. The rats stuck out their tongues and licked their little paws just as they had before. The sugar water was like a sudden jolt of wonderfulness in their gray, dopamine-deprived existence.

But how? If dopamine equaled pleasure and Berridge took do-pamine away, why were these rats able to experience pleasure? And if the rats were able to experience pleasure from food, why did they need to be fed through a feeding tube? None of it made any sense.

Berridge changed tactics again. Instead of wiping out dopa-mine, he cranked it up—big-time—by inserting electrodes in their brains. Now getting the rats to eat was easy. They were vora-cious, eating triple the normal amount. This, however, just made things fuzzier. Despite their gorging, the rats' outward display of enjoyment didn't budge. Sometimes, it appeared to diminish. The rats would sit there stuffing their faces but would open their mouth in a gape, as though to say, "I can't stop eating but this food is awful."

It was a difficult time to be Kent Berridge. The whole world believed that dopamine was pleasure, and there was young Kent, grappling with how it might be all wrong. For years, his research was all but ignored. He has a crisp memory of attending the an-nual meeting for the Society for Neuroscience, and the arctic re-ception he received. These meetings are like sales conventions for science. Researchers present their latest findings on glossy posters with charts and graphs, which they try to sell to their skeptical colleagues. Berridge was standing in a long row of presenters, all of whom had new, cutting-edge data on dopamine. A group of senior scientists made their way down the row, nodding sagely at experiments that confirmed what everyone already knew: dopamine was pleasure. Then they got to Kent Berridge. "Their faces would glaze, and they'd take a few steps backward," Berridge recalls. "They didn't want to get trapped in a discussion with this crazy person."

Evidence, however, is evidence. And evidence that dopamine wasn't pleasure kept pouring in. When patients suffering from Parkinson's disease were given drugs that boosted dopamine, they would do the strangest things. A retired carpenter began sorting his tools and then chopped down a tree for no good reason. An accountant eagerly dismantled his fridge. Elevated dopamine caused patients to go on shopping sprees, take drugs, or gamble— they had a particular inclination for slot machines and scratch cards. Others would pester their wives for sex, masturbate, visit prostitutes, or binge-watch pornography. Yet, what appeared to be indulgences weren't at all indulgent to those doing the indulging. The patients insisted they derived no enjoyment from their peculiar acts. Like Berridge's rats gagging on food they couldn't stop eating, these dopamine-fueled binges never seemed to deliver any actual pleasure.

Berridge turned his thoughts to brain zapping. Combing through the research on pleasure electrodes, he noticed that brain zapping made people do things that *appeared* enjoyable, but no one ever came out and said that it was. For example, a sixty-six-year-old woman who had been depressed for the previous forty-five years was struck by a sudden desire to go bowling.

"This would be quite pleasurable," she said. The sixty-six-year-old woman wasn't sitting there feeling great *at that moment*. The pleasure was off in the distance—something to look forward to.

One study, from 1963, said of one patient "It was as if he were building up to sexual orgasm," but then added, "He was unable to achieve the orgiastic endpoint" and that "this futile effort was frustrating at times and described by him on these occasions as 'a nervous feeling.'" Does that sound like pleasure? Berridge went back to the case of B-19, the depressive, drug-using homosexual, and discovered that B-19 was never quoted—not even once—as saying he felt good.

It took nearly a decade, but Berridge eventually put the pieces of the puzzle together. Pleasure, he discovered, wasn't one thing. It was two. It comprised two different brain systems that were independent but connected. The first is something like a missile tracking system. It becomes aware of the desired target, it tracks and monitors the target, and it goes after the target. If you rev up this system, through brain zapping or drugs, the target becomes extra-desirable, and a person, or a rat, will work extra-hard to obtain to it. If you turn the system down, the world becomes drained of enticement, and the pursuit of pleasure has all the force of a feather landing on concrete. This is the system that runs on dopamine.

Dopamine is incentive. Dopamine is motivation. Dopamine is excitement. Dopamine is *Go!* Dopamine is craving. It is, quite simply, desire. But it is a deep and visceral kind of desire, a primordial urge that is separate from rational thought. Berridge calls it "wanting." Not all desire is "wanting," which is why Berridge always writes the word using italics or quotation marks. The desire for world peace, he says, is not "wanting." "That's not a dopamine thing," he explains. But craving a glass of water after a long run on a hot day is very much a dopamine thing.

It is even possible to "want" something the rational mind expressly does not want—to smoke cigarettes that could give you cancer or to eat a fudge brownie even though you just ate an entire microwave pizza. "Wanting" does not even have to be conscious. If you flash an image of a topless woman at a heterosexual middle-aged man for three one-hundredths of a second, the middle-aged man will not have any conscious memory or awareness of having seen a topless woman. But a brain scanner will reveal a little surge in traffic on his dopamine highway.

But there is one thing "wanting" is not. And this, Berridge found, was the second half of the pleasure puzzle. He calls it "liking." "Liking" is the impact moment of pleasure. "Liking" is payoff. "Liking" is enjoyment. "Liking" is what happens when the sugar water splashes in the rat's mouth. If you think of pleasure as a dinner, "wanting" is the moment you become ensnared by the food's delectable aroma, and "liking" is the moment you put a bite of that food in your mouth and you think, *This is good.*

Most important of all, "liking" is not a dopamine thing. It has its own brain circuitry. It runs on a different set of neurotransmitters that trigger opioid receptors. It is as different from "wanting," neurologically speaking, as a car's windshield wipers are from the windshield itself.

Berridge's many failed experiments began at last to make sense. When his rats were deprived of dopamine, they did not "want" to eat, but nevertheless were able to "like" a squirt of sugar water. And when dopamine was cranked up, their desire to eat raged out of control even though it began to feel unpleasant.

It was as though a chasm had opened in the middle of Michel

Cabanac's "quest for pleasure." There was the quest, and there was the object of that quest. They were two different mental states. It's obvious if you think about it. You *want* to eat a cookie. Then you eat the cookie and *enjoy* it. Perhaps the best evidence that "wanting" is not the same as "liking" is that we so often get disappointed. We want something, we get it, but then we don't like it.

Yet, differentiating these two mental states is often far from clear. "Wanting" and "liking" operate in a continuous blur. A pie can be so good "you can almost taste it"—this is called anticipatory "liking." And when you take that first bite of pie, you want to take a second. The two states can rage simultaneously, as though one has spilled over into the other.

There is a good neurological reason for this. The part of the brain that "likes" is embedded in the part of the brain that "wants"—an island of enjoyment, you might say, amid a sea of desire. These two brain circuits, furthermore, talk to each other constantly. "Liking" fires status updates to "wanting," and "wanting" pays attention. The more you "like" something, the more you come to "want" it. And if you begin to dislike something you formerly enjoyed—an oyster that gives you food poisoning, for example, or a sitcom that stops being funny—you stop "wanting" it. It's a remarkable system. It works.

BUT WHAT if it doesn't always work? If "wanting" can be uncoupled from "liking" in a laboratory—like that time Berridge got rats to gorge on food they didn't enjoy—maybe that can happen in real life? This was the first question Berridge asked after his breakthrough discovery. To answer it, he turned to the most notorious example of pleasure gone wrong: addiction.

In the mid-1990s, there were two competing theories of addiction. The "negative reinforcement theory" held that addicts took drugs to make the pain of withdrawal go away. The pain of withdrawal is, no doubt, real. But there was much this theory could not explain. For example, some drugs, such as certain antidepressants, cause withdrawal yet are not addictive. It is also possible to alleviate the symptoms of withdrawal in an addict, but this does nothing to reduce his or her desire for drugs. There were cases of addicts who had gotten clean and hadn't experienced the pain of withdrawal in years, but would suddenly and tragically relapse.

Then there was the "positive reinforcement theory," which held that drugs are addictive because the feeling of euphoria they produce is irresistible. It makes sense on the surface—the whole point of using drugs is to get high. But addicts themselves outright contradicted this view. Drugs, they reported, lost pleasure with overuse—heroin users, for example, would spend decades chasing that first life-changing high but would never again attain it. Addicts know better than anyone else that the cause of their misery is the drug to which they are addicted, but they go out and abuse that drug anyway. There is also the perplexing matter of nicotine. Cigarettes don't make anyone feel "euphoric." The first time people smoke, they often become nauseated and sometimes vomit. Yet cigarettes are, nevertheless, addictive. People crave them.

Craving. That was addiction's distinguishing attribute. Addicts relapsed because of craving. Addicts deliberately harmed themselves because they were overcome by craving. Sensible and highly functional people smoke, which is well understood to cause disease and early death, because they crave cigarettes. Addiction wasn't about basking in a euphoric state. Addiction was a magnetic pull, as though someone had turned up the sensitivity on pleasure's missile tracking system. Addiction wasn't caused by too much "liking," as everyone always thought. Addiction was a case of too much "wanting."

Berridge and his coinvestigator, Terry Robinson, called their theory "incentive sensitization." You can think of it as the temptation-overload theory of addiction. It's not the high that does addicts in. It's the *desire* to get high, even though that desire doesn't actually deliver the high they so badly want. The theory would go on to change our understanding of substance abuse. For years to come, scientists would scan the brains of humans and rodents alike and find that repeated drug taking causes predictable spikes in dopamine "wanting" that would erupt like solar flares.

After decades of confusion and frustration, there was now a shred of insight as to why addicts seemed set on destroying their lives. Drugs turned the brain's motivation system—the system by which the brain acquires the necessities of life—against itself. And Kent Berridge, the weirdo who was formerly avoided at conferences, would go on to receive the award for distinguished scientific contribution from the American Psychological Association.

NONE OF it had anything to do with food. For more than a decade, Berridge was sure that his research on addiction bore no relation to disordered eating, obesity, or weight gain. Drugs are totally unlike food. Heroin, for example, crosses the blood-brain barrier and binds to "liking" receptors in the brain. Food does nothing of the sort. Sushi isn't more intense if you snort it, and serious chocolate lovers don't inject it directly into their veins. The pleasure of food is all in the sensing. Drugs sensitized the brain, but food did not. Berridge was so confident in this belief that in 2009 he wrote an article dismissing the very idea that obesity had anything in common with his theory of addiction.

A year later, he changed his mind after reading a paper on binge-eating disorder. Binge eaters, Berridge learned, were struck by thoughts of food, even when they weren't hungry. Before eating, they would be overcome with anticipation—classic signs of revved up dopamine. Another study found that adolescent girls with obesity experienced a surge in "wanting" when they saw a picture of a chocolate milkshake, but drinking the chocolate milkshake produced an oddly blunted pleasure response—too much "wanting," not enough "liking." It was starting to sound like addiction.

Another curious piece of evidence appeared. These surges in dopamine "wanting," it was found, could even *predict* weight gain. The cravings, in other words, came *before* the weight gain. One study found that youth at risk for obesity were highly reactive to food stimuli long before they became obese. "In other words," Berridge says, "exactly the right time to be a *cause* and not a consequence of the eventual weight gain." Another study, this one at Dartmouth College, asked forty-eight first-year female students to view a series of images that included a lighthouse, a plate of pancakes covered in syrup, and a naked woman and man in a steamy sexual embrace. The women who experienced the biggest surges in "wanting" at the sight of the pancakes went on to gain more weight. (The women who reacted more strongly to the steamy sexual embrace would go on to have more sex.) A mere picture of food, and the upwelling of desire it produced, could predict weight gain months in the future.

The data paint an utterly different portrait of obesity than the one we know. As with addictive drugs, the food problem isn't fueled by an overindulgence in pleasure, it is fueled by the *desire* to obtain that pleasure. The obese are not selfish pleasure-seekers, as everyone has long presumed. They are instead caught in a vortex of craving. They suffer from a critical dysfunction between two brain circuits. Life with obesity is a kind of cruel prison. To eat is to experience raging bursts of desire followed by an underwhelming dribble of pleasure.

It is a paradigm-shifting insight. And at its heart we find a new and more difficult question: What could cause the metabolically brilliant human brain to malfunction so badly? If the epidemic of obesity is caused by an inflamed desire to eat, why is that desire raging out of control?

PART III

Nutritive Mismatch

How Sweet It Is

Dana Small was eleven years old when she knew she wanted to study the brain. Six years earlier, her mother had developed epilepsy, and Small watched as a woman she'd known to be quick-witted and brilliant struggled to get out of bed in the morning. "That's what sparked my interest in the fragility of consciousness," Small says, "which is what led to the brain."

In 2001, she received her PhD from McGill University, after conducting one of her first and most famous experiments. In it, she gave subjects Lindt chocolates to suck on as their brains were being scanned. The scans revealed that with each successive chocolate, pleasure—or "reward value," as the study called it—diminished. The parts of the brain that were brought to glowing life by the first chocolate became more and more dim. The study, published in *Brain: A Journal of Neurology*, was a breakout success. To this day, Small remembers Wolfram Schultz, one of the world's most prominent neuroscientists, telling her that it was the most comprehensive study yet of motivation in humans. Since publication in 2001, it has been cited around twelve hundred times by other scientists exploring the nature of pleasure, not to mention by an untold number of jour-

nalists who use it as proof of humanity's hardwired and dangerous love of sweetness.

Despite the widespread acclaim, Small often found herself
unsure of what the experiment actually showed. Was sweetness
simply a superficial pleasure that diminished with continued exposure, the way a song can become boring when overplayed? Or
was something deeper going on? Was the brain's opinion of those
chocolates influenced by signals it was receiving from the body
and computations it was making about its needs?

It would take years, but those thoughts eventually crystallized,
sending Small down a twisting experimental path that would lead
to the biggest finding of her career.

IT BEGAN in 2008 at Yale University, where Small had become
a professor. Next door to her office, a Brazilian neuroscientist
named Ivan de Araujo had been running some odd-sounding experiments with mice that were "sweet-blind"—they had been genetically engineered to lack the ability to taste sugar. Araujo then
fed them, of all things, sugar.

Araujo was interested in "post-ingestive" effects. Recall Michel Cabanac's experiment back in 1970, which found that sugar
water only extinguished appetite if it was swallowed—if people
spat it out, their hunger would persist. That meant sugar's biological interaction with the human body went beyond the tongue.
A message, it seemed, was delivered to the brain that said, "Sugar
obtained—cancel hunger." If the sugar water was spat out, however, no such message was sent. This was what led Araujo to do
something as seemingly pointless as give sugar water to mice who
were incapable of tasting sweetness.

The mice were put in cages with three sippers. One was filled with water, another filled with sugar water, and a third one with even sweeter sugar water. The mice, being sweet-blind, had no idea which was which, so they fumbled between dispensers, licking them all equally and randomly, oblivious of sweetness of the liquid flowing down their tiny gullets.

But only for a little while. After six days, the mice's behavior was no longer random. They were deliberately drinking sugar water. They consumed it with same frequency and in the same quantity as mice who were not sweet-blind. Somehow, the "blind" mice knew which sipper was which. Their little brains figured it out.

Araujo also measured the exact patch of mouse brain that did the figuring, a nugget of gray matter called the dorsal striatum. And the brain chemical at work was—drum roll—dopamine. But in this case, dopamine wasn't triggering "wanting." Instead, it was keeping a running tally of the energy contained in the food the mice had consumed. With time, dopamine did enough bookkeeping that deep in the rats' brains, predictions were formed, such as *sipper on the left = calories.* When those mice became hungry, "wanting" kicked in, compelling them to the sipper with calories, which they drank from, all the while not tasting a thing.

As far as the quest for pleasure goes, it was yet another lopsided event. Araujo's mice "wanted" calories and ingested them from the sweet sipper until "wanting" turned off. But their desire was never quenched by enjoyment. "We didn't see the classic liking signs," Araujo says. There was no paw licking, no gleeful tongue-poking. The mice were like whiskered little robots.

Araujo followed this study up with one that was even stranger. This time, he used regular lab mice and put them in cages with two sippers—one contained water mixed with sucralose, an artificial sweetener, while the other contained an extremely bitter chemical called denatonium benzoate. The bitter sipper, however, was configured in such a way that when a mouse drank from it, a little burst of sugar would be injected into its stomach. Araujo thus "rewrote" the rules of taste. Sweetness now indicated no calories, while bitterness did the opposite. Once again, the mice behaved like intelligent energy-seeking robots. They gave up on the sweet but ultimately useless sipper and opted instead for the wincingly bitter taste of the denatonium benzoate, as though magnetically drawn to the calories it provided.

The rules of taste, it seemed, weren't carved in stone (confirming what Howard Moskowitz had already witnessed in Bangalore in 1975). Sweetness may be hardwired, but it is just a cue, a label, whose meaning can be overwritten. The system was adaptable and intelligent. If bitterness and sweetness swapped roles, a mouse could reprogram itself on the fly. The stomach wasn't some dumb and unfillable pit—it was an active participant, sending information to the brain, information that was recorded with each meal and used to make predictions about future meals.

The brain doesn't just keep tabs on how much sugar enters the mouth or how much sugar winds up in the stomach. It even keeps track of *what happens* to that sugar. In another mind-bending experiment—he has a reputation for them—Araujo gave mice a drug that blocked sugar from being turned into energy. The mice tasted the sugar and it was sensed in the stomach, but if it couldn't be used as fuel, sugar it lost its magnetic pull. What the brain ultimately cares about isn't how food tastes. It cares whether food is *useful*.

*   *   *

ARAUJO'S FINDINGS brought Small's thoughts back to her Lindt chocolate experiment. What was it, exactly, she wondered, that she'd witnessed in the brains of her chocolate eaters? Was it a simple attraction to sweetness fading in those brain scans? Or was it a deeper attraction to calories that was fading to black?

It is a fine and good question, but how do you answer it? Araujo had the luxury of using mice that were incapable of tasting sweetness, which meant their attraction to calories was based purely on post-ingestive learning. People, alas, have tongues that can sense sweetness. Small could offer human subjects all the sugary candies or drinks in the world, but there would be no way of knowing if their urge to eat was powered by the delight of sweetness or an unconscious drive for calories. How could Small measure in humans what Ivan de Araujo had so exquisitely observed in genetically engineered mice?

This is how: Small created five separate drinks, each with a distinct flavor and color. She then added a precise amount of the artificial sweetener sucralose, so that each drink tasted as sweet as a drink that contained about seventy-five calories of sugar. Finally—this was the key step—she added varying amounts of a chemical called maltodextrin, a simple, high-calorie starch that is tasteless. This allowed her to manipulate the calorie count of each drink while leaving the taste unchanged.

Dana Small had thus created a little arsenal of drinks that tasted equally sweet, but each carried a different energy payload: 0, 37.5, 75, 112.5, and 150 calories. Small gave samples of the drinks to her test subjects, so that their brains could "learn" the caloric value of each. Next, she scanned their brains as they sampled each beverage. If she detected any differences in "wanting" areas of the brain, she knew it would have to be due to the calories and not the sweetness, because the drinks, remember, all tasted equally sweet.

It was ingenious. Dana Small had found a way to separate calories from sweetness in human test subjects, and now she would be able to measure which was doing what. Everything about the experiment was perfect except for one thing: it didn't turn out at all the way she expected.

Small had anticipated that the highest-calorie drink would trigger the biggest surge of blood flow in the dopamine highway. A hundred and fifty calories are more biologically useful, after all, than 0 calories, 37.5 calories, and so forth. Yet, it was the 75-calorie drink that generated the clearest spike of brain activity.

What was going on? If calories were driving the desirability of the drinks, then the 75-calorie drink should have produced less motivational oomph than the 150-calorie drink. But it produced more. If calories had nothing to do with desirability, why would a 75-calorie drink be more desirable than a 0-calorie drink? It made no sense.

The more Small thought about it, however, the more the results began to come into focus. What came into focus, specifically, was a single number: 75. The drinks had all been designed to taste as though they had 75 calories worth of sugar. And it was the 75-calorie drink that produced the biggest brain response: 75 and 75. Was this more than just a coincidence?

To answer that question, Small moved from the brain to the body and measured how each of the drinks was metabolized. It was a simple experiment. Subjects would enter the lab, consume one of Small's drinks, then be connected to a machine called an indirect calorimeter, a device that analyzes the heat a person's body produces and from this can estimate the quantity of calories being burned. It is a textbook response called the thermic effect of food. When the body takes in calories and uses them, it generates heat as a by-product, the same way the engine of a car heats up after it's been running. The more calories a person consumes, the greater the thermic effect.

That, at least, is what the textbooks say. But that is not what Small found. She can vividly remember the day her laboratory assistant showed her the initial results. "It blew my mind," Small says. "I knew right away we were onto something new and exciting."

A few days earlier, a female test subject, a woman in her twenties, had consumed the 75-calorie drink and was subsequently connected to the indirect calorimeter. On cue, her body produced a little plume of heat, indicating that the 75 calories were being burned.

Days later, the same woman returned and drank the 150-calorie drink and, once again, was connected to the indirect calorimeter. There should have been a gradual uptick in heat production. Her body should have produced more heat with the 150-calorie drink than it had with the 75-calorie drink. And then Small's lab assistant shared data that seemed almost impossible: the indirect calorimeter measured nothing. It was as though the twentysomething woman had not consumed a single calorie. The "metabolic response," as Small put it, "was flat."

The findings were so odd Small did the experiment over again, but the results did not change. Over time, a distinct pattern had emerged: when people consumed the drinks in which the sweetness and calories were not in sync, the calories those drinks delivered would not be properly metabolized. Small calls the phenomenon "nutritive mismatch." The maltodextrin would splash into their stomachs, where enzymes would convert it into sugar, and the sugar would be absorbed into the blood. But then, oddly, it wouldn't get burned. Like a film of gasoline floating atop seawater, the sugar just circulated in the blood. When the drinks were "matched," on the other hand—when the level of sweetness correctly indicated the caloric payload—the calories were burned as expected.

Small's research journey had taken a ninety-degree turn. By attempting to discern what made sweetness desirable, she had unexpectedly discovered something more fundamental. Sweetness wasn't just an enjoyable taste sensation. It was a metabolic signal, the first spark in a string of biochemical processes by which sugar is turned into energy. Sweetness was like the trumpeter at the castle gates. It heralded not only the arrival of calories, but the specific quantity and began making arrangements for how they would be used.

When sweetness and calories match, it all hums along: calories are burned, the brain registers it, and the brain remembers. But when there was an unexpected variance between what the tongue sensed and what the stomach received, the entire metabolic process seemed to shut down. "It's like the system just threw up its hands," Small says, "and didn't know what to do."

Did nutritive mismatch have long-term consequences? This question prompted Small's next study, which looked for a hallmark of diabetes called insulin sensitivity, a condition in which cells no longer respond properly to this crucial hormone. Small tested drinks with sugar, drinks with no calories, and drinks where sweetness and calories were mismatched. Once again, the results were as amazing as they were alarming. The mismatched drinks—and only the mismatched drinks—impaired insulin sensitivity.

Finally, Small fed mismatched beverages to teenage boys and girls. This was a particularly relevant investigation because adolescents are in a period of heightened body and brain development and so have an outsize calorie appetite, which is one reason teens drink a lot of sugary beverages. The study had barely even begun when Small and her team drew blood from three subjects and discovered, to their great alarm, that two had already become prediabetic. An ethics board reviewed the results and deemed the health risk to be so great that it would be unethical to continue.

IF THE thought of unmetabolized blood sugar and prediabetic teenagers alarms you, there is more bad news. Those drinks didn't even taste good. The highest-scoring beverage inched above "like slightly" but didn't crack "like moderately." Small's brain scans showed plenty of cerebral action, but "liking" wasn't invited to the party. It was "wanting." Her beverage-drinking volunteers from the New Haven area were like those sweet-blind mice—drawn to consume drinks they did not particularly enjoy.

It makes one wonder: Where did this idea that obesity is an excess of pleasure come from in the first place? This is the root of a long-standing stigma against fat people. They indulge themselves to excess. They are too selfish to say, "I may want more, but enough is enough."

Scientists typically refrain from making such judgments (except about other scientists), but the prevailing view among the white-lab-coat crowd is a less guilt-laden version of that stereotype. Obesity, the experts keep telling us, is caused by an over-abundance of "highly palatable foods"—pizza, ice cream, chicken fingers, cheeseburgers, and the like. Lately it has become fashion-able to refer to such foods as "hyperpalatable," the idea being that these ultraconcentrated wallops of sweet and salty calories deliver a hit of bliss so strong it "sensitizes" the brain, just like addictive drugs.

It is the latest iteration of the Hungry Ape Theory. As theories go, not only is it easy to believe, it is comforting, too. It lets us lay the blame on the greedy food industry for stuffing us full of calories while delivering scientific assurance that it's not our fault because we are biologically programmed to succumb to these irresistible confections.

If only life were that simple. It is easy to paint calories as humanity's enemy, which perhaps explains why we have gleefully been doing so for decades. But to malign the lowly calorie is to fundamentally misunderstand the evolutionary story that brought our species into existence.

Several million years ago, the brains of our evolutionary ancestors were roughly a third the size they are now. Brains are energy hogs. They burn lots of calories. Having a small brain meant our ancestors could survive on a low-calorie, fibrous plant diet. They spent much more of their time foraging and eating, compared to us, and they had long, slow-moving digestive tracts that were needed to extract nutrients from this kind of diet.

As humans evolved, however, a trade-off took place. Our brains got much bigger, while our guts got smaller and faster. (This theory is known as the "expensive tissue hypothesis.") A big brain paired to a small gut meant we had to upgrade to food that packed a bigger caloric punch: fatty meat, nuts, seeds, grains, sweet fruit, and the like. Four entirely separate populations of humans—one in Europe, two in Africa, and one on the Arabian Peninsula—evolved the ability to digest milk into adulthood, giving them the lifetime ability to consume one of the few sources of fat blended with carbs found in nature.

Eating such a calorie-rich diet brought with it a great advantage: time. We spent less of the day obtaining food. We saved countless hours of needless chewing. Instead, we began to do the things that make us human: we fashioned tools, erected structures, shared stories, created myths, and played games. We invented cooking, which made our rich, easy-to-digest food even easier to digest.

Calories made humanity possible. Calories are what fueled our big brains. Our calorie-rich diet didn't reinforce the compulsion to eat, it released us from a food-gripped existence. It gave us the time to do big brainy things. Just because we require calories does not mean our basic programming compels us to overconsume them, for the same reason that requiring oxygen does not compel us to perpetually hyperventilate. Yes, it may be advantageous to carry extra calories in time of famine, but this assumes an overly simplistic view of our evolutionary past. Out there in "nature," carrying extra body weight brings serious, even deadly, disadvantages, as Daniel Nettle from Newcastle University has argued. To the evolving primate, greater body mass means slower acceleration and a sacrifice in the ability to change speed or direction quickly. Back when we were prey—when our ancestors were habitually eaten by big cats, hyenas, pythons, and even eagles—our ability to nimbly start, stop, and turn was crucial for survival. To a predator, a fat human was not only easier to spot and easier to catch, it made for a bigger, better meal. To the prey that we hunted, a fat human was easier to evade and out-run. Carrying too much fat also increases the likelihood of injury and death due to "the forces and loads involved in maintaining a larger body." To put it in the simple arithmetic of evolution-ary fitness, being unnecessarily fat didn't increase an individual's chances of passing on their genes. It reduced them.

As we became more advanced, there were even more reasons to refrain from overindulgence. Food had to be shared with other members of the tribe, then the village, then the town, especially with children, whose dependence on adults for resources lasts an eternity compared to other species. We began sharing food with wolves, which became dogs.

Eventually, we reached one of the great landmarks in our species' development: we figured out how to store food. Eleven thousand years ago we stockpiled grain in purpose-built facil-ities that kept it dry and free from rodents so we could eat it weeks and months after harvest. Ancient Egyptians collected honey from apiaries and stored it in clay pots. Five thousand years ago, Native people living on the Great Plains smashed bison bones into pieces and boiled them in steaming vats fash-ioned from animal hides. When the rendered fat rose to the top, they scooped it off and blended it with dried meat and berries to make a carb-, protein-, and fat-rich calorie bomb called pem-mican.

This innovation brought with it an incredible leap forward in energy efficiency. When calories are stored as fat, a great deal of energy is wasted just hefting all that extra weight around. But when food energy is preserved outside the body—in clay pots, in granaries—you achieve far greater efficiency.

Storing food, however, also required an essential mental capability: the ability to resist eating it. Ancient Native Americans didn't sit there for days at a time stuffing themselves full of pemmican until none was left. They feasted after the bison hunt, but they retained the ability to set aside enough for the brutal winter yet to come. There was an evolutionary fitness advantage in being able to say, "I will eat this later." If we didn't have that ability—if we really were slaves to an unrelenting appetite for calories—the human species would have died off long ago.

All of which leaves us with the following paradox: Why were humans generally able to resist vastly overconsuming calories up until about fifty years ago? In Dana Small's research, we at last see the beginning of an answer.

Ever since organisms began sensing food as it entered their body, the information gathered was reliable. This is why the ability to taste evolved in the first place. No creature has forty minutes to sit and digest a meal so its brain can determine if it has had enough to eat. It is much more efficient to take a reading as the food comes in. The ability to sense food is so crucial, in fact, that more DNA is devoted to systems that sense the taste and flavor of food—the nose and the mouth—than any other part of the human body. Tasting food engages more gray matter than any other activity.

This system, as we have seen, is designed for accuracy. But it evolved in an environment in which food provided the senses with accurate information. Dana Small's research shows what happens when that changes—when the food we eat tells the brain a nutritional lie. The system fails. Calories enter the blood but are not burned. "If sweeteners are disrupting how carbohydrates are being metabolized," Small explains, "then this could be an important mechanism behind the metabolic dysfunction we see in diets high in processed foods."

To make matters even worse, we appear to be entering a golden age of nutritive mismatch, and ironically, it is in large part due to the widespread panic over sugar. To a food company, nothing could make more sense than blending sugar with artificial sweeteners. Both the calories and the amount of "sugar" appearing in nutritional info panels decreases, but the sweetness stays constant and the food or drink remains as tasty as ever. Creating nutritive mismatch is, simply, good for business. There is mismatch popping up all over the beverage aisle—in Gatorade Lower Sugar, Dr Pepper TEN, Nescafé Sweet & Creamy Ice Java, and AriZona Low Carb Caution Performance Energy Drink. In Britain, it is no longer possible to purchase full-sugar versions of Sprite, Schweppes Indian Tonic Water, and Dr Pepper anymore. They're all a blend of sugar and artificial sweeteners.

This is happening to food as well. You can bring home a bag of Thomas' Whole Wheat English Muffins from the supermarket, which contain sugar, but also sucralose. Dannon Light & Fit Greek Yogurt contains sugar as well as stevia. Sara Lee Delightful Honey Whole Wheat Bread, Fiber One Honey Clusters cereal, Nesquik No Sugar Added, Reduced Sugar Craisins, Hershey's Lite Syrup—all textbooks cases of sweetness that isn't matched to the calories. An Orange Fanta in New York City has 160 calories. The British version has 63 calories. Even mismatch is mismatched, geographically.

So here, at last, we have found a fundamental aspect of food and eating that has changed: the sensed nutritional value. For as long as humans and their ancestors existed, the taste of a calorie matched the energy it delivered. In the span of just a few decades, that has changed. Calories don't "mean" what they used to.

We are tampering with the very way the brain perceives food, and the implications are still revealing themselves. We know nutritive mismatch is harmful to the human body, that it disrupts metabolism on an elemental level. Here then is an even more disturbing question: What is its effect on the brain?

7

Not Losing Isn't Everything.
It's the Only Thing

Losing feels worse than winning feels good.

—Vin Scully, retired sportscaster

On March 21, 2003, a software engineer from Los Angeles inserted a $100 chip into a Megabucks slot machine at the Excalibur Casino, in Las Vegas, Nevada, and hit a jackpot totaling $39.7 million. To this day, no slot machine has surpassed that stupendous payout. It was, statistically speaking, an event of extraordinary rarity, like the meteor impact that wiped out the dinosaurs.

Slot machines are what's known as a negative equity game—the odds are designed to favor the house. Most people know this. What most people don't know is that the house only keeps a small percentage of what it takes in—most of the wagered money is returned as winnings. This is part of what makes slot machines so exquisitely unpredictable, which, as we shall see, is what makes them so irresistible. But make no mistake: these games are rigged, and no strategy or technique can turn things to the player's advantage. The best you can hope for is to win early and win big and then never play the slots again. But people play them anyway.

Gambling, especially problem gambling, is a lot like obesity in that way. Both are self-destructive, often ruinous forms of pleasure seeking. Problem gamblers wish they could stop gambling the same way problem eaters wish they could stop eating. The comparisons do not end there. Gambling may be the best window we have into understanding why people eat beyond their needs. At the most basic level, both behaviors appear fueled by the same internal drive: to gain. The eater wishes to gain food, while the gambler wishes to gain money.

The truth, as we shall see, is more strange. What looks like an intense desire to gain is actually something quite different: an attempt to avoid a loss. We humans have an aversion to losing. We fear, abhor, and detest it. The drive to avoid losing is so deeply entrenched in our psyches that its mind-altering effect is similar to taking drugs. The mere whiff of a loss cranks up the brain's "wanting" circuits to such a degree that it compels us to do irrational things. Casinos are experts at turning this inborn trait against us. But so is the food environment. And what ignites our fear of losing—what causes us to eat to the point of sickness—is nutritive mismatch.

IN THE late nineteenth century, a Russian scientist noticed his dog had a habit of drooling. At first it seemed that food was what caused the dog to drool, but one day the Russian scientist observed that the dog would drool even if there was no food. Over time, it became apparent that the drooling was spurred by the sound of footsteps, which indicated to the animal that it was about to be fed. This got the scientist thinking. He started turning on a metronome—a device that clicks to help musicians keep time—before serving the dog dinner. At first, the clicking did nothing. But over time, the clicking made the dog drool as predictably and reliably as the footsteps. The dog didn't need to see, smell, or taste anything. The sound of clicking was enough. It is what has come to be known as a conditioned stimulus.

You have probably heard of the scientist, Ivan Pavlov—a brilliant but also peculiar figure who had a savage temper and, at one point, harvested the digestive liquids of dogs and sold them as medications. Pavlov had a near obsessive interest with the fluids secreted by the digestive tract. Among all the fluids he studied, however, one held a special place of honor: drool. It was a "psychic secretion." The mere thought of food could get a dog drooling.

We call this kind of response Pavlovian. A simple association such as "clicking = dinner" is one of the most basic ways animals, and people, make sense of the world. It is a form of learning, but it isn't like math or remembering how to spell words like *isthmus*. It is learning that we *feel*. It comes from deep down. When you are driving at night and see a glowing restaurant logo in the distance and experience a sudden urge to stop and eat, it happens automatically. You don't have a choice in the matter.

How strong are these mental associations? How intense is the feeling of "wanting" that something as neutral as a click or a restaurant logo can produce?

Psychologists long believed it came down to reliability. For example, if ringing a bell sometimes predicted dinner but sometimes did not, its motivating effect was considered medium. But if a bell always and dependably predicted dinner, that bell became almost like a substitute for food itself. For decades, this was the standard belief in psychology. It turned out, however, to be wrong, and we have pigeons to thank.

In the late 1960s, two scientists at McMaster University, in Hamilton, Ontario, began studying the Pavlovian responses of these generally uninteresting birds. Each pigeon was placed in a special box with a key that could be depressed. The key would be illuminated by a white light, and a moment later a little hatch would open, revealing food. At first, the pigeons didn't notice the key, then the hatch would open, and they would perk up and peck the grain. In time, the pigeons seemed to grasp some connection between the illumination of the key and the delivery of food. Some pigeons developed a peculiar habit: they would peck the key. The key, remember, did not cause the food to appear. It was just a sequence—key is illuminated, food hatch opens. But the pigeons pecked the key anyway.

Almost a decade later, a British psychologist named Bob Boakes was curious if rats shared this same predilection. He repeated the McMaster experiment, replacing the key with a lever. The lever didn't do anything other than form part of a sequence—lever is illuminated, pellet drops. Rats, Boakes discovered, were a little bit like pigeons, but not completely. Just as some of the pigeons pecked the key, some of the rats began nibbling the lever. The other rats headed straight for the food hatch, waiting for it to open.

Boakes decided to drill deeper into the rat psyche. He performed the experiment again, but this time he made a crucial alteration: now when the lever was illuminated, the food sometimes dropped, but sometimes did not. The illumination of the lever, to use technical language, became an "uncertain" cue. The order was random and impossible to predict, but odds worked out to fifty-fifty.

If rats had any sense at all, you'd figure they would give up on the unreliable lever and focus on the food pellets. What good, after all, is a lever that's wrong half the time?

But that's not what the rats did. The rats flocked to the lever. They would press it and nibble it, almost as if they were trying to fix whatever had gone wrong. Uncertainty didn't reduce the lever's allure as everyone had always presumed. Instead, it cranked it up. A predictable lever is not exciting to a rat. An unpredictable lever, now *that* was something worth checking out.

AROUND ABOUT the same time, two very different psychologists made a similar finding. They weren't studying food or why humans overeat. They were interested in gambling. Amos Tversky and Daniel Kahneman, a now-legendary Israeli duo, wondered what it was about gambling that caused people to make irrational decisions.

It had long been assumed that people gambled for a simple reason: to acquire money. The chances might be slim, but the thought of a huge reward made it seem worth the risk. This "get money" theory of gambling was compelling—everyone dreams of winning big—but there were aspects of gambling the theory could not account for. For one thing, it is well-known that people often place bets for tiny rewards. Some people play poker with pennies, for example, which does not result in a significant acquisition of money. People who are extraordinarily wealthy will enthusiastically put down $10 on a football game. A rich person does not benefit from winning $10. So why place the bet? And why do it eagerly?

That was the thing about gambling. It *felt* a certain way. It stirred an excitement that went beyond money. For example, if a worker is offered a holiday shift that pays triple, he might be happy to take it, but the prospect does not excite him—he doesn't tell his friends or kick off the shift with a big steak dinner. High-paying work, such as corporate law or dentistry, is considered conventional and banal. In that sense, gambling didn't look anything like an opportunity to make money. Just thinking about gambling gets people excited.

The answer took Kahneman and Tversky years to figure out. It would revolutionize the study of economics and lead to a Nobel Prize. But it did not come from analyzing calories or measuring dopamine or studying rats. It came from examining risk.

Kahneman and Tversky wanted to know how humans "intuitively" handled risky situations—how they reacted when faced with a choice with an uncertain outcome. They carried out their research by handing out little booklets filled with simple questions and asked respondents to fill in whatever answer popped into their heads. Here is an example Kahneman uses in his book *Thinking, Fast and Slow*:

Problem 1: In addition to whatever you own, you have been given $1,000. You are now asked to choose one of these options: 50 percent chance to win $1,000 or get $500 for sure.

You probably chose the $500. That's what most people choose. Here is another example.

Problem 2: In addition to whatever you own, you have been given $2,000. You are now asked to choose one of these options: 50 percent chance to lose $1,000 or lose $500 for sure.

This time you probably decided to take your chances on losing $1,000.

That was the problem. According to the prevailing view, decisions of this sort were governed by whichever option brings people the greatest expected value or gain. Problem 1 and Problem 2 should therefore each have the same answer, because the outcomes are identical—you can either choose to be $1,500 richer for sure or take a fifty-fifty shot at going for $2,000 with the risk that you might only end up with $1,000.

The two questions, however, generated different answers, even though the only thing that made them different was the wording.

Here is another Kahneman-and-Tversky classic:

Problem 3: An 80 percent chance at $4,000 or $3,000 for sure.

Problem 4: An 80 percent chance at losing $4,000 or a $3,000 loss for sure.

It's clear that Problem 4 is the "mirror image" of problem 3. One choice is about *getting* money and the other is about *losing* it, but the probabilities are identical. And if people made decisions in the "rational" way they were supposed to, the answers would be simple to predict. For Problem 3, the "rational" choice would be an 80 percent chance at $4,000, because it is, mathematically speaking, more valuable than $3,000. (It has an "expected value" of $3,200, which is to say that if you took this option a whole bunch of times, you would average $3,200.) Similarly, an 80 percent chance at losing $4,000 has an expected value of –$3,200, so a "rational" person would choose the sure loss of $3,000.

But people overwhelmingly give the "wrong" answer to both questions. When it came to gaining money, they would take the safe bet of $3,000 for sure. But when faced with losing money, 92 percent of people opted to take an 80 percent chance at losing $4,000—a bad bet.

What was driving this seemingly irrational behavior? It wasn't a desire to *gain* money. It was the desire to avoid a *loss*. The mere thought of a loss, the researchers found, has a warping effect on how people handle uncertain situations.

When Kahneman and Tversky published their findings, it forever changed our understanding of human behavior. Economics, the discipline founded on the notion that people are rational decision makers, had to grapple with the fact that they often are not. The human animal wasn't some clinical thinker, a calculator made of flesh and blood for whom the world was filled with probabilities. Life was a hodgepodge of possible gains or losses to which people reacted automatically, emotionally, and sometimes irrationally. You lunged at some prospects, while others were so repellent you took reckless gambles to avoid them.

With this newfound insight into human nature, behavior that once seemed needlessly self-destructive began to make sense. For example, when problem gamblers are on a losing streak, rather than cease gambling—the sensible thing to do—they often begin taking larger and more dangerous bets. The phenomenon is known as loss chasing. Just like people who eat well beyond their needs, gamblers enthusiastically do something the whole world knows they ought not to. It is not because the gambler is a depraved fiend. He doubles down because what he craves, more than anything else, is to get out of the hole, and a big, high-stakes bet is the only way to do it. To walk away means accepting the loss—a bitter pill to swallow. Thus, the normally risk-averse human, who ordinarily craves certainty, opts to do something stupid. "A person who has not made peace with his losses," Kahneman and Tversky wrote in 1979, "is likely to accept gambles that would be unacceptable to him otherwise."

Kahneman and Tversky had hit upon the same pattern of behavior as Bob Boakes and his lever-pressing rats. An uncertain outcome didn't decrease motivation—it ramped it up.

In 2003, the Cambridge neuroscientist Wolfram Schultz published the results of an experiment that not only crisply illustrates this baffling tendency, but links it to the world's most famous brain chemical. In his experiment, monkeys were shown simple pictures that *might* or *might not* result in a reward of concentrated black-currant juice. A picture of a box was followed by no juice. A picture depicting three bars meant juice was a sure thing. If the monkeys were shown an X, however, they might get juice or they might not. The X indicated uncertainty. All the while, Schultz measured "dopamine activation" in the monkeys' brains after each picture was presented. The box, it comes as no surprise, triggered the lowest surge of dopamine—it indicated no reward. The three bars, however—which indicated a definite reward—registered an equally low dopamine response. A certain reward was just as unexciting as no reward. It was the *uncertain* cue—the X—that triggered the largest surge in dopamine.

However "irrational" this may seem, it is by design. The brain, as we have seen, monitors the energy we take in and the energy we expend. It does this for a good reason: energy is necessary to survive, thrive, and reproduce. The world, however, is full of surprises. So the brain keeps track. Constantly. It tabulates what happened in the past so it can predict what's going to happen in the future. If a behavior results in a gain, it gets entered in the logbook. Same for a loss.

When the brain faces an uncertain situation, however, it has a default setting, and that setting is to ramp up motivation, to work harder—to strive for *more*. Why? Because evolution favors winners, not losers. Deep in our ancestral past, the organisms that responded to uncertain situations by working harder stood a greater chance of avoiding a loss, which made them more likely to thrive and reproduce than their brethren who shrugged in the face of risk.

This behavioral strategy is so deeply etched into our psyches that we aren't even aware of it. Uncertainty doesn't feel uncertain—it doesn't plunge us into stretches of brooding indecision. It *excites* us. An uncertain prospect—a slot machine, a scratch card—pulls us in. We cave to impulse. It ignites "wanting."

Some scientists see uncertainty as a grand unifying theory of the brain. According to this view, the brain is something like a giant prediction engine, constantly comparing the present with the past so that it can prosper in the future. Numerous scientific journals are devoted to this apparently obscure subject, including the *Journal of Risk and Uncertainty*; the *International Journal of Uncertainty, Fuzziness and Knowledge-Based Systems*; the *Journal of Risk Research*; *Risks*; the *Journal of Risk and Insurance*; and *Risk Management*. Extremely intelligent people spend entire careers studying nothing but risk, uncertainty, gains, and losses.

And if you think for one moment that you are beyond uncertainty's reach, that you possess the all-seeing wisdom or strength of mind to overcome humanity's dread of losing, think about buttons. Think, specifically, about buttons that don't always work.

Here are three examples:

1. The walk button at busy intersections.
2. The close-door button on elevators.
3. An elevator call button.

Not one of these buttons is dependable the way a light switch or a faucet is dependable. Walk buttons are so unreliable, people wonder if they are even connected. Many elevator close-door buttons are not connected—they are dummy buttons that can only be activated by maintenance or emergency personnel. An elevator call button, by comparison, sends out a signal, but it has no control over the arrival of an elevator.

Now consider how you *feel* about these buttons. Do you press the walk button once and wait patiently for the light to change? No, you jab at it incessantly. The same way you repeatedly press the elevator call button even if someone else already pressed it. And when you finally step into the elevator only to discover that the door-close button is uncooperative, you punish it with a staccato burst from your hotheaded index finger. These buttons call out to you—*Press me*—and you eagerly oblige. You are, at that moment, experiencing "wanting." The uncertainty of these buttons has elevated your motivation.

Do you press other buttons this way? When you walk into a room, do you punch the light switch on with a pronounced intensity? Or do you flick it, mindlessly and gently? If you want an elevator to take you to the eleventh floor, do you stand there relentlessly poking the 11 button until you reach the eleventh floor? Or do you press it just once? The answer is once. Why? Because the 11 button is reliable. The outcome is certain, so you don't work as hard to attain it. It's boring.

Uncertainty, on the other hand, is so universally enthralling that we set up organized bouts of it. We create rules. We buy tickets and congregate by the thousands so that we may all sit and experience a roller-coaster ride of edge-of-your-seat risk. We call these events games. We may think games are about winning and losing, but those are just outcomes. Games are driven by the excitement of not knowing what's going to happen next. The slimmer the odds, the more exciting the match. No one is roused by the prospect of watching a pro basketball player play one-on-one with a retired podiatrist. We like nail-biters. The excitement reaches its peak when the odds approach fifty-fifty.

So now for the big question: Does uncertainty have the same effect with food as it does with money? The answer is a resounding and disturbing yes.

For gerbils.

A scientist at the University of Stockholm performed an experiment in which he placed eight of these perky-eared critters in a "superabundant" food environment. One bowl was fantastically crammed with seeds—it contained more than a thousand. Next to it was another bowl with two hundred seeds—still a huge amount—but in this bowl, the seeds were mixed in with sand, so a gerbil would have to use its paws to carefully extract a seed if it wanted to munch one. Halfway through the experiment, however, the gerbils woke up to a very different world. One food bowl was empty, containing only sand. The other was filled with a paltry hundred and fifty seeds, and they were mixed with sand. Conditions kept changing. One day there were more seeds, the next there were fewer. And the bowls were never in the same spot. The gerbils' "food environment" had gone from being certain to uncertain.

The effect on their eating was clear: when food became unpredictable, the gerbils ate more. When meals were solidly predictable, they ate less. It is the little details of this experiment, however, that stand out. For instance, when food was superabundant, the gerbils ignored the big bowl. They seemed to derive some satisfaction from pulling seeds out of the sand, even though doing so took more time and effort—not what you'd expect from creatures "wired to get fat." When the situation became uncertain, however, this predilection evaporated. The gerbils went into a kind of panic and headed for whichever bowl was more "profitable."

There is one additional detail that is both the most astonishing and the most alarming. The gerbils never faced anything close to an actual food shortage. During "uncertainty," there were fewer seeds available and they were always mixed with sand, but there was still much more food than the gerbils were capable of eating. As with gambling, what motivated the gerbils wasn't some in-built urge to acquire—it was the prospect of losing.

From a distance, the behavior seems rash and irrational. Why gorge when there's still plenty to eat? But it's easy to envision why this sort of response might make good sense in nature, where it would probably be wise to start storing fat at the first sign of a food shortage, not once it's gone. "The possible need for storing," the gerbil-feeding scientist wrote, "has to be calculated at each moment." It was as though uncertainty whispered a thought in those gerbil brains: *Eat, because tomorrow you might lose.* The gerbils were pulled into one of nature's oldest games. And they ate.

ARE PEOPLE like gerbils? Does the mere thought of not having enough food make us eat beyond our needs? This idea occurred to a Boston doctor named William Dietz in 1993 while treating a female patient who weighed exactly the same as him. Dietz was forty-six and weighed 175 pounds, which is what he weighs today. His patient was seven.

Bill Dietz was running what was, at the time, one of the nation's few obesity clinics and had seen cases far more severe than this one. What caught his attention, however, was a comment the patient's mother made. Dietz had recommended eating more fruits and vegetables—the added bulk, he'd hoped, would take up more space in the young girl's stomach, leaving less room for the calorie-dense foods that were contributing to weight gain. The mother told Dietz the family lived on welfare and food stamps, and after the rent was paid, money would get so tight that nothing would be left to spend on food. At these times, the mother served her daughter rich, filling meals such as chicken wings, beans, and hot dogs. If she served pasta, she would add extra butter or oil.

The situation seemed paradoxical. A literal shortage of available calories was matched by an unhealthy excess of stored calories. Maybe, Dietz thought, the mother was consciously trying to ward off hunger by serving rich and satisfying foods. But it occurred to Dietz he was witnessing a deeper behavioral response. Maybe, as Dietz wrote in the journal *Pediatrics*, "obesity may represent an adaptive response to episodic food insufficiency."

His article, aptly titled "Does Hunger Cause Obesity?," kicked off a boom in scholarship. Two decades later, almost everyone is at least vaguely aware there is often a relationship between obesity and people's level of education, their income, or their racial background. A study done in King County, in Seattle, for example, found that the strongest predictor of obesity was the value of a person's home—the lower the home value, the higher the likelihood of obesity. The three poorest states—Mississippi, Arkansas, and West Virginia—are the three states with the highest rates of obesity. This link between wealth and body fat has also been observed in Luxembourg, Australia, Sweden, France, and England. Even in Italy, the elevated rate of obesity in the south—the supposed land of olive oil and fish—is explained by the region's relative poorness compared to the north. Scientists in Singapore recently found that if a person just imagines him- or herself interacting with a wealthier, better-educated, and more respected peer, he or she becomes more sensitive to the energy density of beverages. It is as though at some elemental level the brain understands low status to be a loss, one that warrants a compensatory gain in calories.

Yet, this connection between wealth and body weight still seems fuzzy. Poverty, you see, is no guarantee of obesity. It just raises the risk. So scientists have focused the lens more tightly and measured "food insecurity"—not knowing where the next meal is coming from, or if there is even going to be a next meal. Here, the connection with obesity becomes even stronger. Scientists call this the insurance hypothesis of obesity. Food insecurity is perceived as a threat to future well-being. So we ward off the threat of hunger and starvation by eating more.

From a distance, it may seem maddeningly self-destructive

that people chronically short of money would eat food they can barely afford and clearly don't need to eat. But if you think of human beings as animals who are programmed on a deep level to respond to uncertainty in predictable ways, this is just what you would expect.

This hidden aspect of our nature brings unintended consequences. For example, parents often restrict access to unhealthy foods, such as cookies, in an effort to reduce the amount their children eat. Studies have found that this strategy often backfires, bringing about the opposite result. Restricting food elevates its allure. Cookies become a fixation. Children complain about the unfairness of the situation, and then when the cookie jar finally appears, they lunge for it. Mothers who tick yes to statements like "I have to be sure that my child does not eat too many high-fat foods" or "If I did not guide or regulate my child's eating s/he would eat too many junk foods" have daughters who are more likely to eat even when they are not hungry. None of these children face anything close to the threat of starvation or even missing dinner. An unreliable cookie supply results in exaggerated cookie desire.

This is the reason the poor tend to be fatter, even though they have less money. It is not because they are unintelligent or self-indulgent. It is because, however rational we may believe ourselves to be, the appetite follows its own evolutionary logic.

Yet, this only still explains one small part of the mystery. Food insecurity is not the sole underlying cause of obesity. How could it be? Millions of financially secure people, who have never been poor or known food insecurity, are nevertheless overweight or obese. Their situation seems more paradoxical. Why would people who can afford more food than they need nevertheless eat as though they cannot?

The answer is, once again, explained by our ingrained response to uncertainty and loss. But in this case, it is not the prospect of eating that has become uncertain, as was the situation with Bill Dietz's seven-year-old patient and those Swedish gerbils. Food itself is now coaxing the brain into a disturbed state of "wanting." The reason we can't stop eating, we will see, is simple. Uncertainty has been baked into the taste of the food we eat.

8

Creamfibre 7000

On October 25, 1949, a patent for "alginate ice-cream stabilizing composition" was awarded to the Kelco Corporation. Alginate is a compound found in seaweed. According to the patent, it improved the shelf life of ice cream—it let you leave ice cream in the freezer longer without unpleasant ice crystals forming. Since then, we have learned that alginate's talents are numerous. It can thicken mayonnaise and salad dressings and keep the foamy froth on the top of a beer perfect. But if you go back and read the original patent filed by the Kelco Corporation, you will find that stabilizing ice cream came with another benefit: it imparted "a desirable body and smooth texture to the frozen product." It made ice cream taste richer than it actually was.

Over the decades to come, commercial ice cream makers learned that alginate, along with a long list of other stabilizers, emulsifiers, and thickeners, meant they could cut back on costlier ingredients such as cream and eggs. It is one of the thousands of food technology breakthroughs that have shaped what and how we eat today.

If you subscribe to the Hungry Ape Theory and believe that the human appetite is dim-witted and in need of strict governance, these discoveries appear almost like gifts from God. Consider saccharin, which was discovered in 1879, and which gave humanity the gift of unlimited sweetness with no calories. It is hard to imagine a better deal.

A deal that good, however, is almost always too good to be true.

Think back to Dana Small's mismatch experiment. There were five drinks, all identically sweet but each containing a different amount of calories. What sticks out is the bodily consequences of nutritive mismatch—sugar getting into the blood, sugar not getting burned as fuel, adolescents becoming prediabetic, and so forth.

The brain wasn't sitting idly by minding its own business as all this went on. It was keeping track, as the brain always does. Each drink knocked on the front door—the mouth—and said, "Sugar! Energy!" But only one of those drinks was telling the truth. The others told the mouth one thing and the stomach something else. The sensory cue that is sweetness became shrouded by uncertainty.

This sensory tampering is a recent development. Our species, *Homo sapiens*, has lived on this planet for about three hundred thousand years. Sugar is older, and the ability to sense it stretches back hundreds of millions of years. Bacteria can sense sweet. So can cockroaches, worms, and mice, and so could our earliest ancestors, who subsisted on fruits and leaves in ancient tropical forests. What we call "sweetness" is information, a reading about one of nature's oldest forms of calories.

We changed that. We took a reliable predictor of calories and turned it into a "maybe." We now live in a world where sweetness *sometimes* indicates lots of calories, *sometimes* indicates some calories, and *sometimes* none at all. Sweet taste has become like a slot machine. You push the button, but you don't know what you're going to get. Ice cream, whose taste once reliably predicted its calorie load, has become, year by year and additive by additive, uncertain. The "prospect" of a rich and creamy bowl of French vanilla could mean:

(a) 290 calories
(b) 174 calories.

What does this do to the brain? It comes down to, once again, odds. A single hit of saccharin isn't going to induce the eating equivalent of loss chasing. It is when the relationship between calories and sweetness becomes sufficiently chaotic that you would expect the brain to infer the threat of losses and respond accordingly.

A scientist at Purdue University named Susie Swithers presented this very condition to laboratory rats. All of them were fed a sweet-tasting rat chow along with yogurt. One day, the yogurt tasted sweet, and the next it did not. But the yogurt wasn't sweetened the same way for all the rats. For half, the yogurt was sweetened with saccharin, and for the other half it was sweetened with ordinary sugar. Both groups thus lived equally sweet lives, but for one group that sweetness always indicated calories, and for the other it *sometimes* indicated calories.

If you subscribe to the idea that sugar is addictive, as has become fashionable, then the rats that got more sugar should have eaten the most food and gained the most weight. That is not what happened. The rats who were intermittently given saccharin gained the most and ate the most. For them, the relationship between sweetness and calories went from a solid "yes" to "maybe." It is an echo of that gerbil experiment back in Stockholm. Lots of food isn't what makes rodents overeat. It is uncertainty that cranks up "wanting." And fake sweetness is one way to create uncertainty.

THE WORRY that artificial sweeteners may be harmful to our health is anything but new. They have been studied almost as long as they have existed. And the results are all over the map. In randomized controlled trials—experiments in which one group of people is fed artificial sweeteners and another group is not—it usually, but not always, looks as if artificial sweeteners may help people lose a tiny amount of weight. But when scientists observe people in the real world over long periods of time who use artificial sweeteners versus those who do not, they find that those who consume artificial sweeteners are at higher risk for weight gain, heart disease, metabolic syndrome, and diabetes. Not long ago, a group of European scientists gathered up all the research examining the relationship between artificial sweeteners and body weight and examined it for clues. They found that in the experiments that tested a "learning paradigm," where the caloric meaning of sweetness was altered, artificial sweeteners more dependably resulted in weight gain. In other words, perhaps some specific recipe or set of circumstances puts "wanting" into overdrive.

Exactly what that recipe might look like is a deeper question. It may be that different and seemingly disconnected forms of uncertainty can collectively gang up on "wanting." For example, merely exposing a teenage girl to artificial sweeteners may not, on its own, trigger an eating response. But if that uncertainty is added to the stress of a recent parental divorce along with the stress of enrolling at a new school, the effect may well be different.

All that said, we know this sensory tinkering is having an effect. When scientists scan the brains of people who habitually consume artificial sweeteners versus people who do not, they find differences. They see more activity in the dopamine circuits that compute "reward value" and that get fired up by uncertainty. In our brilliance, we think these wonder substances fool the brain. But the brain is too smart for these simple chemical dodges. The brain knows something isn't right and it responds.

Artificial sweeteners are far from perfect imitations of sugar. The chink in their armor has always been their artificialness. "Linger" is one problem—their cloying tendency to taste sweet for too long compared to sugar's pleasing fade-out. A mild but detectable bitter taste is another issue, as is the lack of mouthfeel. Sugar, on the other hand, adds a syrupy richness to liquids and makes them taste more filling.

These subtle differences between artificial sweeteners and sugar may help our brains distinguish one from the other. Nevertheless, food scientists have been hard at work eliminating these faults. Food companies now add special compounds called bitter blockers to eliminate the bitter issue. Mouthfeel is imparted by adding tiny amounts of soluble fiber to a beverage. And that cloying linger can be dealt with by adding a little salt. Year by year and additive by additive, the taste of fake sugar is getting closer and closer to the real thing.

Another less well-known class of sweeteners aims for partial fakeness. Compounds such as xylitol, isomalt, and maltitol, for example, are twice as sweet as sugar, calorie for calorie. These don't deliver sweetness with no calories, just *fewer* calories. They are members of the family known as sugar alcohols, they tend to cause diarrhea, and Americans collectively consume about three hundred and sixty-five thousand tons of them every year. A more recent addition to the happy gang are positive allosteric modifiers—chemicals that alter perception itself by modifying sweet receptors on the human tongue so that the signals they send become amplified and sugar becomes an exaggerated version of itself. You can think of them as the fun-house mirror of nutritive mismatch.

Then there are fake fats, a family of high-tech food additives that is as large as it is unknown. Unlike the makers of artificial sweeteners, the makers of "fat replacers" have had the good sense to lurk in the shadows, and their chemical wizardry has, by some miracle, evaded the scrutiny of nutrition professors, dietitians, and food activists. There is one famous exception: olestra. Discovered in 1968 by scientists researching baby food, this miracle substance looked, smelled, tasted, and even cooked like fat. Incredibly, it contained *zero* calories. It did everything fat did but with no funny aftertaste, no bitterness—nothing. Olestra was so superbly fatlike that you could fry potato chips in it, which is what Frito-Lay did, marketing low-calorie versions of Doritos, Tostitos, Ruffles, and Lay's under the WOW moniker. In the end, though, olestra's camouflage was its undoing. Enzymes in the gut that bond with fat molecules didn't react with olestra and let it sail by, and it arrived at the end of its digestive journey as pristine as at the beginning, causing a constellation of unpleasant symptoms, the most famous being "anal leakage."

Before it was laughed off the market, Susie Swithers did an olestra version of her artificial-sweetener experiment at Purdue University. One group of rats only ever ate potato chips fried in full-fat vegetable oil, while another group got regular chips one day and olestra chips the next, thus experiencing caloric uncertainty. The rats that got the full-calorie chips ate less and gained less. The rats that got olestra half the time—the ones that lived in an *uncertain* food world—ate more and were fatter. Once again, injecting uncertainty into the caloric "meaning" of a taste sensation cranked up calorie intake.

Does the same thing happen with people? There is one curious study from back in 1992, before olestra had even been approved by the FDA. In it, one group of men ate regular biscuits made with full-fat fat, while another group of men ate biscuits made with olestra, and a third group ate biscuits made with even more olestra. After breakfast, the men given the most olestra had consumed 316 fewer calories than the men who downed the regular biscuits. But after lunch, dinner, a snack, and breakfast the following morning, that gap had dwindled to almost nothing. Within mere hours, their brains not only registered that something wasn't quite right with those rich, fatty breakfast biscuits, but, on cue, "wanting" cranked up to close the gap. How did it close the gap? By seeking carbohydrates. It was as though their brains recognized that fat had become uncertain and so sought certainty in carbs.

The fake-fat story does not end with olestra. There are more far more fake fats than there are fake sweeteners, and unless you have spent the last three decades living as a hunter-gatherer, you have eaten many of them. You may have even eaten some today. In 2017, America ate more fat replacers than any other country in the world. In 2022, the United States will consume nearly $500 million in fat replacers, and the global appetite for these brain-fooling products is set to exceed $2 billion. That is quite a lot of fake fat, considering it can cost all of ten cents to replace the fat in a serving of yogurt.

If you are wondering why you have never heard of fake fats, the answer is that the industry prefers it that way. When I contacted one of the leading researchers in the field, a scientist who works at a publicly funded university and whose name is attached to scores of publications, he informed me that he refuses to speak to journalists as a matter of principle.

There is, however, another reason most of us are in the dark about fake fats. They are complicated. The human tongue is forested with taste buds that contain taste receptor cells. Each of the basic tastes—sweet, salty, bitter, sour, and umami—has its own taste receptor. Fat, too, has its own receptor, but, puzzlingly, it doesn't seem to deliver a distinctive taste signal to the brain. Exactly what it does remains uncertain. (Some scientists believe these cells sense rancid fats.) What is certain, however, is that fat does not have a characteristic taste of its own, not the way salt tastes salty or sugar tastes sweet. Fat is more of a feeling. Fat is slippery. Fat is smooth. Fat is rich, moist, and thick and coats the tongue. This is because fat is sensed by the mouth's touch receptors. We possess an extreme talent for sensing the textural qualities of fat. Whipped cream feels different from custard, which feels different from butter or cream-cheese icing. Fat becomes light and sumptuous when you aerate it. It makes foods deliciously crispy when you fry things in it, and it also carries many of the flavor chemicals that make food delicious. Fat isn't so much a tough act to follow as an impossible one.

Well, almost impossible. If you look hard—and the food industry has looked very hard—you can find chemicals that mimic some of the properties of fat, just not all of them. One of the first was discovered in 1979 when a food scientist working for a large Canadian brewing company tried turning whey (the liquid left over after making cheese) into a gel. His attempt resulted in a substance that had the gelatinous qualities of egg white but crumbled like Styrofoam. Most important, it tasted fatty—like cream cheese or cheesecake. It was a landmark moment in food history. A cheap liquid cheese by-product could be made to mimic the way fat stimulates nerve endings in the mouth, but at a fraction of the calories. This miraculous effect was caused by tiny balls of protein—40–50 billion of them in a single teaspoon. The substance, which is technically referred to as microparticulated whey protein concentrate, was sold to NutraSweet, which refined it and launched it in 1988 as an industrial food additive called Simplesse. Simplesse could turn a teaspoon of margarine, which normally has 36 calories, into an 8-calorie low-fat spread or shave 153 calories from a small bowl of ice cream. With Simplesse, "a creamy garlicky commercial salad dressing had all the richness of ordinary salad dressings," as the *Chicago Tribune* raved at the time. The richness was an illusion created by technology. The brain sensed creamy fat coming in, but all the stomach got was tiny protein balls.

Simplesse tastes creamy, but it's a lousy thickener. To solve that problem, you can turn to a product called Slendid, a high-ester pectin. "Bulking" is achieved with products such as CrystaLean, Lorelite, and D-LITE. Mouthfeel and "flow" are delivered by Avicel, Methocel, and Solka-Floc. Creamfibre 7000 may sound sci-fi, but it was designed as a "fat replacement in muffins." It makes water taste like fat.

Names such as Methocel, Beta-Trim, or Lycadex sound painfully corporate and do little to arouse the palate. These are the industry brand names, the cheesy monikers for which the creators of processed food have a peculiar affinity. You'll never find one on an ingredient panel. Simplesse goes by "milk protein" or "whey protein concentrate," which makes it sound as if it came from a farm. According to its brochure, Genutine "can help you create a range of gelatin-like textures for desserts, confectionery and dairy systems," while Genugel "is used to create rheological profiles ranging from free-flowing liquids to thixotropic liquid gels and self-supporting solid gels with a wide range of textures, setting temperatures and melting temperatures." But you know them, if you know them at all, as "carrageenan." One of Creamfibre 7000's many attributes is its "clean label." It shows up on the ingredient panel using an absurd but technically correct alias: "citrus fiber," which sounds not only healthy but as if it might prevent bowel cancer.

Each of these products is a bit fatlike on its own, but not one is anything close to the real thing. However, when you add them together—one for bulk, one for flow, one for creaminess—magic happens. The simulation of fattiness becomes so effective you don't know it's happening. The food business refers to these mixtures as "combination systems."

SOME PROCESSED foods fool the senses even when that isn't their intent. The 1950s saw the invention of "modified" starches. We extracted carbs from foods like potatoes and corn and chemically altered them to enhance their food-processing applications. We then began putting these stealth carbs in everything from salad dressings to pie fillings. Today, food processors can choose from a list of emulsifiers, starches, and gums so long it would have to be spiral-bound. Thanks to this handiwork, ice cream takes longer to melt, the cocoa doesn't separate and form a dark layer in chocolate milk, and frozen foods don't release dreadful puddles of water as they are heated.

Maltodextrin, the miracle starch Dana Small used in her experiments, may be the most fantastically mismatched substance in all of creation. It can add body to fruit juices and forms the powdery base for potato-chip seasoning, yet it can also function as a fat replacer in dressings and spreads. Some forms of maltodextrin are flavorless, while some taste sweet. It was created in 1967. Before that, maltodextrin-induced nutritive mismatch did not exist.

Then there are "flavorings." Long before the boom in artificial sweeteners and artificial fats, the flavor industry exerted a transformational effect on food, thanks to a device called a gas chromatograph, which became commercially available in the 1950s. The GC, as it is known, made it possible to capture and identify the flavor compounds that give foods their vivid character. One of the first moves industry made was to identify flavor compounds in butter and add them to margarine. Artificial berry flavorings, which had long tasted painfully fake, soon became astonishingly real. The mouth told the brain, "Berries!"—but all the stomach received was a little jumble of chemicals.

We were not designed for this. Nature endowed us with the ability to sense the finest gradations between foods, but those differences, as subtle as they might be, meant something. If a piece of pork was fatty, not only could you see the fat, you could taste its mouth-filling richness. Meaty foods tasted meaty. Starchy foods like potatoes, pasta, and rice tasted soft and comforting. The flavor of food always had a fixed relation to what that food was. The senses delivered accurate, reliable information. Packaging was an act of biology, not marketing.

Food isn't like that anymore. Starting around the midpoint of the last century, wave after wave of food-processing innovations have created a divergence between the nutritional content the brain senses as it consumes food and the actual nutrients that arrive in the stomach. Sucralose, gums, carrageenan, modified starches, methylcellulose, stevia, flavorings, saccharin, microparticulated protein, Solka-Floc, maltodextrins. Each new molecule adds another little dose of uncertainty.

In the span of decades, the taste of food went from highly certain to highly uncertain. A condiment as simple as mayonnaise has gained a level of nutritional unpredictability reminiscent of quantum physics. To know how many calories are in a tablespoon of mayonnaise, you need to know which mayonnaise you are eating. A tablespoon of Hellmann's Organic Mayonnaise has a hundred calories. Hellmann's Extra Creamy Mayonnaise tastes richer, yet also comes in at a hundred calories per tablespoon. Hellmann's Real Mayonnaise, meanwhile, has ninety calories, while Light has thirty-five, and its Low Fat Mayonnaise Dressing has fifteen. It sounds like one of Dana Small's experiments, but it is not an experiment.

Fat replacers have made their way into every imaginable food. You can find them in salad dressings, gravies, sauces, soy milk, pasta, shepherd's pie, cookies, cake, croissants, cheese, yogurt, sour cream, ice cream, milk shakes, candy bars, chocolate, cream, and processed meat. Some fat replacers are organic.

The "whipped light cream" McDonalds uses to top its Frappés and hot chocolate is a lower calorie confection of cream, nonfat milk, mono and diglycerides, natural flavors and carrageenan.

The "white whipped topping" at Tim Hortons, the Canadian doughnut chain, contains hydrogenated vegetable oil, dextrose, sodium caseinate, modified cellulose, polysorbate 60, microcrystalline cellulose, natural flavor, soy protein concentrate, polyglycerol esters of fatty acids, and xanthan gum. But no actual cream. Uncertainty.

Oikos Triple Zero Blended Greek Yogurt tastes creamy, sweet, and fruity but contains no fat, no added sugar, and no fruit. Halo Top Blueberry Crumble ice cream stimulates sweet receptors with stevia and erythritol (a sugar alcohol), aroma receptors with natural flavors, and mimics the sensation of fat with milk protein concentrate, whey protein concentrate, organic carob gum, acacia gum, and organic guar gum. Uncertainty.

What is all this uncertainty doing? Exactly what a behavioral economist would predict. It is producing a vigorous drive to avoid losses. Consider a few of the more noteworthy landmarks in the recent history of American food. The Big Gulp, supersizing, breaded chicken wings, the 20-ounce plastic Coke bottle, the BK Triple Stacker, stuffed-crust pizza, KFC's Double Down, the 540-calorie Ultra Caramel Frappuccino, Cinnabon's 1,080-calorie Caramel Pecanbon, Cold Stone's 1,740-calorie Reese's Chocolate Peanut Butter Dream milkshake, or the 2,590-calorie Crispy Honey Chipotle Chicken Crispers & Waffles at Chili's.

Not a single one of these foods represents a cultural high point in sensory pleasure. These foods are about quantity. That's why they feature verbiage such as *double*, *triple*, *ultra*, *super*, and *dream*. They are the eating equivalent of loss chasing. No matter what any scientist tells you, these foods are not "hyperpalatable." They do not represent the apex of eating pleasure. They just seem that way to people caught in the grip of "wanting." What they are is "hypercraveable."

* * *

HERE IS one of the most amazing facts about America's food problem. Americans consume more calories than the Italians or French and yet somehow spend less than half as much time eating. We are like those panic-stricken gerbils in Stockholm. We stuff our faces as though famine is around the corner. For so long, the cause of our disturbed eating has been invisible. That has made us cling—often religiously—to false and idiotic theories.

The picture is at last becoming clearer. The thing that changed—the event that energized "wanting" and created this artificial, inescapable hunger that has ensnared so many of us—is nutritive mismatch. For the first time in the history of our species, the information the brain senses about food has become consistently unreliable.

The food environment is now something like a calorie casino. The threat of losses makes people behave in self-destructive ways. We were not born to be fat. The problem is we are being goaded into a game we cannot resist. And it is killing us.

PART IV

The Help That Hurts

9

Why Does Food Taste Good, Anyway?

When Johann von Goethe crept into that horse-drawn carriage on that foggy September morning more than two hundred years ago, he directed his coachman toward Italy. No one is quite sure why. To those who knew him, his departure seemed rude and abrupt. Just days before, he was "jolly and carefree," and then, just like that, he bolted. His friends accused him of being un-German and a deserter. In truth, Goethe had been planning his escape to Italy for months. He invented an alter ego under which he would travel and sent out sums of money to collect during his journey, so as not have to carry an unduly large amount. On the first leg of the trip, he implored the coachman to hurry. "My lust to see this land," he would later write, "was overripe."

What was the object of that lust? It was not pellagra, or some benevolent interest in the well-being of peasants. His chance encounter with those sick women and children in Veneto is hardly mentioned. In a diary totaling more than 122,000 words, the disease garners a total of four sentences.

Was it Goethe's interest in architecture that drew him south? Or that his father had made a similar trip during his own youth? Or was Goethe, like so many travelers, drawn to Italy for the food?

In his first diary entry, Goethe wrote, "I am longing for grapes and figs." In the first two weeks of travel, fruit is mentioned no fewer than eleven times. Its quality, he believed, would improve the farther he moved south.

The Italian countryside did not disappoint. As Goethe descended from the Alps, the hills were covered in trees bearing the olives and the figs he had been dreaming of. He spent a night in a town called Torbole, which was so poor the locals covered their windows with greased paper because they couldn't afford glass. The food, however, moved him. For dinner, Goethe ate trout fillet, the flavor "delicate and excellent," but his "real delight" were the figs and pears served for dessert. Two days later, Goethe toured a local vineyard, and his guide sent his fifteen-year-old scrambling up a tree to "pluck me the best fruit."

At a farmhouse south of Palermo, Goethe sipped wine and watched as two traveling noblemen dismounted their horses, cut the tops off some thistles growing by the side of the road, peeled off the rind, "and devoured the inner part with great satisfaction." In a Sicilian town called Agrigento, he spent an afternoon observing a local family make pasta. They kneaded the dough, rolled it into "long pipes," then twisted each piece into an S shape. The resulting dish he described as "the most excellent macaroni." Yet, of all the foods this German visitor ate, the one that left the most indelible mark was, of all things, Sicilian lettuce. He described its flavor as "milky."

It is all recounted in a book called *Italian Journey*, published in 1816 and still in print. The trip left him a changed man. When he returned home after two years—far longer than he had initially intended—a friend complimented Goethe on how slim and tanned he looked. Another thought he seemed newly "sensual."

Goethe planted trees and berries in his garden. In a town of six thousand in eighteenth-century Germany, he managed to procure foie gras, truffles, mussels, chestnuts, salmon, and caviar, which he would serve to guests at grand afternoon dinners. He grew berries, fruit trees, potatoes, and herbs in his garden and raised foreign varieties next to local ones so that he could compare their different flavors.

It is a remarkable turnaround for a man whose life once seemed on the verge of collapse. But this is the absolutely least impressive thing about Johann von Goethe.

Here, briefly, is his story:

At the age of twenty-five, Goethe published *The Sorrows of Young Werther*, a story about a lovelorn romantic who commits suicide. The book was a sensation, shooting Goethe to a level of fame difficult to comprehend even in the pop-culture era. A mania called "Werther fever" took hold of Europe. Men would dress up in outfits identical to that of the novel's main character: custard-yellow pants and a bright blue jacket. Women spritzed themselves with a perfume called Eau de Werther and sipped tea from porcelain cups and saucers featuring scenes from the novel. There were, reportedly, copycat suicides. In England, a young woman was found dead in her bed with *The Sorrows of Young Werther* under her pillow. In Germany, a man clutching a copy hurled himself off a tall building.

Among the book's multitude of fans was the duke of Saxe-Weimar-Eisenach, a kind of microstate in what is now Germany. The duke was impressed by Goethe and invited him to live in the duchy. He bought Goethe a cottage, had it renovated, and named him as an official adviser. The author quickly discovered he possessed another talent: statesmanship. Over time, Goethe would rise to become the most powerful civil servant in the duchy. At his peak, he was in charge of mines and highways, the war commission, and the treasury. He ran the place.

Through it all, the man somehow kept writing. He is Germany's most towering literary figure, and his magnum opus, *Faust,* is considered one of the greatest written works, period. It comes as a comfort, therefore, to learn that Goethe detested pretense. At a puffed-up official dinner at a merchant's home, Goethe took a large painted portrait off the wall, cut the face out of it, then inserted his own face in the opening and sat there, laughing it with up guests. Later that night, he and the duke got drunk and rolled huge barrels of wine down a hillside.

His friend was right to describe Goethe as sensual. When he wasn't searching out great food in Italy, he would duck into churches to see famous paintings. The man bounded from one experience to the next as though his purpose on earth were to prepare a grand report.

Now compare Goethe's indulgences—superb fruit, art, travel, rolling wine barrels down a hill in the middle of the night—to a rat pressing his brain-zapping lever 850,000 times. A psychologist might coldly define both as "pleasure-seeking" activities. Yet they could not be more different. The rat is caught in a spiral of "wanting." The rat desires one thing, and only one thing. Goethe, by comparison, lusted to do things he had never done before. If Goethe could have stepped inside a brain scanner while eating those figs in Torbole, I think he would have lit up the other half of the brain's pleasure system. Johann von Goethe was the crown prince of "liking."

* * *

A SNAKE would never eat a fig. Snakes are carnivores. But if a snake did eat a fig, and if you imagine that snakes could talk, a snake would not comment on its flavor, good or bad, because it is incapable. Snakes have almost no sense of taste.

What snakes are good at is smelling. They have nostrils. As a snake breathes, it samples the air constantly, and if something catches its attention—a scampering field mouse, say—the snake upgrades to more sensitive form of smelling: its forked tongue. The snake sticks out its tongue, oscillates it at ultrahigh speed so it can ensnare odor molecules, then pulls it back in and deposits the odor molecules into a kind of second nose located in the roof of the mouth. A snake's tongue is forked for a reason—the odor molecules captured by each branch inform the snake if prey is to the left or right. Hunting is a rich sensual experience for a snake. But what follows, eating, could probably be compared to swallowing for a human, a necessary physical exertion that delivers little pleasure.

This is by biological design. How a mouse or a frog tastes doesn't matter to a snake. Their sensory system is aimed to detect, hunt, and kill, and that's where it ends. A snake can spend weeks lying in wait for the opportunity to strike at passing prey. Once its prey is dead, however, the snake is in no position to taste it and opt to wait for a bigger, plumper critter. The snake has already expended too much energy. In economic terms, the sunk costs are too high. Taste offers a snake no valuable information, so possessing that sense is pointless.

The system all runs on "wanting." Lying in wait, striking, squeezing prey until it has suffocated—all dopamine driven. A snake's dopamine system is a close match to our own. The motivation circuit is one of evolution's major achievements. It is also an extremely old one, stretching back to around 600 million years ago, to a common ancestor that looked something like a slug. It is, remember, the "getting stuff" system. A slug has to be just as successful at getting food as an eagle or a human. If you don't get stuff, you die.

A snake's eating system can be likened to a thermostat. The system receives an "error signal"—information that something isn't quite right—and moves to fix it. In the case of the thermostat, the error signal might be that room temperature is too low, in which case the thermostat sends a signal to the furnace, the furnace begins producing heat, and the room temperature is gradually restored to its preferred setting, at which point the thermostat cancels the heat signal and the furnace shuts off. But there is no pleasurable sensation for a thermostat as waves of heat gradually raise the temperature. And there isn't for a snake, either. There is no evidence that snakes experience "liking." If snakes had language, there would be no word for *ahhhh*. They are reptilian behaviorists. They spend their lives making urges go away.

It can be hard to wrap one's head around this. Only the cruelest of gods would create an animal incapable of *enjoying* the meal it worked so hard to get. But when it comes to enjoying food, snakes are the norm. The vast, vast majority of creatures get by just fine on the thermostat model. Error signal, "wanting," feeding. The end. The system works and has done so for hundreds of millions of years.

The question we should be asking, therefore, is not "Why don't snakes enjoy their food?" but "Why do we?" Why does "liking" exist at all? If the capacity to enjoy dinner isn't necessary for a snake, why do we have it? Why did evolution deem "liking" a trait worth keeping?

* * *

THE ABILITY to taste what you are eating has benefits. One significant advantage is that you can tell if something is wrong with your food. This is not an issue for snakes because snakes are carnivores and their food is almost never poisonous. Animals that eat plants, on the other hand, face the constant threat of being poisoned. A bright red berry might look plump and juicy and might be full of sweet calories, but it might also be toxic. What saves us from calamity, ultimately, is the tongue. It can detect energy in food by sensing sweetness, but bitterness is often a dead giveaway that a berry or leaf is poisonous.

Tasting food helps an organism get a head start on digestion. The mere sight or aroma of food triggers a burst of stomach acid and a squirt of insulin, known as the cephalic phase. When food enters the mouth, the festival of gastric secretion continues. Tasting carbohydrates releases more insulin, while tasting protein triggers the release of a different hormone called ghrelin. Despite the widespread myth that the taste of food is utterly disconnected from nutrition, the two are inseparable. If that pre-bite cephalic squirt of insulin does not happen, the meal that follows causes something like a temporary case of diabetes—sugar accumulates in the blood and is not properly metabolized. The human organism is a high-performance, fast-running, hot, wet, salty dynamo. You can't just dump in fuel willy-nilly. Each little glob of nutrition needs to be identified so that it may be properly broken down and absorbed. The brain, remember, is hell-bent on predicting, and the tastes and flavors it senses during eating helps it do just that.

The critical role played by taste is best illustrated by the sad yet miraculous case of Tom, a nine-year-old Irish American who, in

1895, burned his throat so badly while eating clam chowder that his esophagus became permanently sealed. Doctors saved him by creating an opening in his abdomen, and for the remainder of his surprisingly long life Tom fed himself by loading food directly into his stomach as cargo is loaded into a truck. Tasting food was now utterly pointless, yet Tom insisted on doing just that. He would chew his food, then spit it into a funnel fitted to a hose connected to his stomach. This apparently pointless act saved his life. Immediately after doctors surgically created the opening in his stomach, Tom remained poorly nourished no matter how much food his nurse or mother inserted in his stomach. One day, the sickly nine-year-old uttered a request: *Let me taste my food first.* He sprang back to good health. More than four decades later, he told doctors that if he didn't taste food before inserting it in his stomach, he'd still be hungry after the meal.

The mouth is a more than a hall of frivolous chewing. It senses important information about food, information that forms the beginning of the long process whereby food is taken in, broken down, and used. But that still doesn't answer the big question: What does any of that have to do with food tasting *good*? If you think about it, the mouth, with its multitude of taste receptors, could fit perfectly into the thermostat model. The mouth could inform the brain, say, that a sweet cookie has arrived. "Wanting" flares as the cookie is excitedly bitten down to nothing, then recedes as satiety is achieved. It would all work perfectly well without even the tiniest spark of "liking." If you could wave a magic wand and grant snakes the gift of taste, that doesn't mean they would enjoy food. For pleasure to take place, specific brain circuitry is required.

So what, then, is the purpose of that circuitry? What use is there in experiencing pleasure when we eat? Why does feeling good feel good?

It is a colossal head-scratcher. The "wanting" system exists to get stuff. Why did the "liking" brain circuit evolve?

It helps, at this point, to stop thinking about food. Forget about insulin and the cephalic phase and all that and just stop thinking, period. Instead, listen to music.

Music is in some ways a better window into the mysteries of eating than eating itself. It is impossible to scan a person's brain as they eat because chewing causes too much head movement and introduces too much "noise." (This is why so much research features liquids—they can be injected directly into the mouth as a subject lies still.) You can, however, scan the brain of a person listening to music, and doing so offers clues about the workings of the brain that would otherwise remain obscured.

Music engages the same "reward centers" in the brain as eating, treating us to the continual cycle of "wanting" followed by "liking." Consider a standard song with verses and a chorus. The first verse catches your attention and primes you for what's coming next. This is "wanting." This is a dopamine moment. The anticipation of the chorus builds, then, on cue, the chorus arrives, and with it a shower of "liking." At its pinnacle of intensity, this phase can induce chills and goose bumps, a state of exhilaration researchers refer to as a skin orgasm. Scientists define the phases of musical pleasure as "excitement" followed by "consummatory" followed by "satiety." Music is a meal you eat with your ears.

There is a simple but dependable way to use music to achieve "liking": set an expectation and follow through. Verse followed by the chorus. Tension, release. It feels good.

Brain imaging, however, shows there is a way to generate

an even bigger eruption of "liking." Instead of simply following through with what is expected, "violate" expectations. Don't deliver what the listener thinks is coming. Catch them off guard with something *even better*, something amazing they didn't expect—a sweet yet aching harmony, or a sudden change of key. The unexpectedness of it jerks us to attention. The physical response—goose bumps and chills—is similar to a fear response. The brain realizes something is amiss. But when the brain identifies that this unexpected thing is a good thing, the *opposite* of a loss, we are upgraded to a higher tier of pleasure. We are left feeling moved, cleansed, purged, and reborn. Music can tear you to shreds and stitch you back together better than new.

In this we find a clue to the purpose of "liking." It is, simply, *quality control*. It tells us if what the getting system got is bad, good, or better than expected. The computational power at work is staggering. When we bite into something—a peach, a pork chop, a chocolate—we can instantly tell not only if it is good or bad, but just where it fits on that spectrum. The ability to enjoy or dislike food is quality computation that you *feel*.

Why did "liking" evolve? For the same reason all traits evolve: because it can give creatures a survival advantage. But not just any creature. For a snake, one meal is very much like the next, nutritionally speaking. Everything the snake needs—the energy, the protein, the vitamins, the minerals—is all contained in the prey it swallows whole. This is the carnivore strategy: get what you need by eating a similar but smaller version of yourself. The strategy ensures quality, so there is little point in sensing it. (This is one reason that carnivores such as sea lions, which like snakes swallow their prey whole, have lost much of their ability to taste.)

Other creatures take a different approach. Instead of eating one thing, they eat lots of things, a feeding strategy known as om-nivory. This is the category we humans fit into. An omnivore gets it all—calories, protein, vitamins, minerals—from many different foods. This seems like a brutal if not impossible undertaking. No single food contains all the necessary nutrients we require to live. Different foods, furthermore, contain different nutrients in dif-ferent amounts. And some foods are poisonous. To make things even more convoluted, the omnivore's needs are an up-and-down jumble—children require more energy per pound of body weight than adults, who themselves have a higher vitamin requirement. Pregnancy throws everything for a loop.

The great food psychologist Paul Rozin called this predica-ment "the omnivore's dilemma." (The famous book by Michael Pollan would come much later.) How did we solve it? With "lik-ing." The mouth tells us what the eyes can't: how sweet, how rich, how salty, how starchy, if it's poisonous, and so forth. You can't tell how good a peach is by looking at it. But you can by biting into it. If it's bad, we spit it out. If it's good, we keep eating. If it's excep-tional, we become lost in its spell.

THERE IS an old theory that states our appetites are "in tune" with our deepest biological needs. As with body temperature and thirst, the thinking goes, what we crave is in lockstep with what we require. If, for example, someone is in need of a particular vi-tamin, they become stricken with a desire for a food that contains it. The idea is called "the wisdom of the body," which is the title of a book by Walter Cannon, who was the chairman of the De-partment of Physiology at Harvard Medical School from 1906 to 1942.

Much has changed in a century. Most of the scientists who study nutrition and eating today believe the human appetite is driven by a lust for calories and bears no relation to our complex physiological needs. If those scientists are right, then animals truly are smarter eaters than humans, despite their smaller brains. Take the goats of Olympic National Park as an example. Despite the park's wildflower meadows and jaw-dropping views, goats never lived here for the simple reason that they could not. The area receives too much rain, which washes life-sustaining minerals into the ocean. (In this sense, it is a kind of inverse Karnataka—too much water, not enough minerals.) That all changed in the 1920s, when hunters introduced goats to the area, thinking it would be a fine place to shoot them. Human visitors also alleviated the park's nutritional shortcomings by excreting urine, which is rich in the minerals that goats need. The goats of Olympic National Park discovered that drinking human urine solved their internal mineral shortage. Like shifty drug dealers, they would sit in wait as hikers relieved themselves in the bushes, then rush in to lap up a liquid we humans find abhorrent. By doing so, they found a way to prosper in an environment where survival was formerly impossible.

A similar intelligence exists in rodents. If certain vitamins become scarce, rats and mice will eat their own feces. This seems the height of nutritional stupidity, but like all animal behavior it has a purpose. The bacteria in a rodent's microbiome can synthesize the very vitamins the rat or mouse requires, and its own excrement thus provides the nourishment the original meal lacked.

Animals, it would appear, are gifted eaters. And if you consult the history books, you would make the same conclusion about humans.

In the year 1602, a Spanish expedition was heading north from what was then New Spain along the coast of California when the crew became sick. It started with a kind of generalized but extreme body pain so intense you couldn't even touch a victim's pajamas without causing agony. The skin erupted in purple dots "larger than great mustard seeds." Gums started swelling and teeth loosened so that "they move while moving the head." Death, when it came, could be disarmingly abrupt. "They die all of a sudden, while talking," the voyage's priest wrote in a diary. When the expedition finally pulled into Mazatlán, all that could be heard on deck was a dismal chorus of groaning and prayer.

Soon after reaching port, a group of soldiers rowed out to a nearby island to dispose of the mounting pile of corpses. A corporal suffering from this mysterious disease noticed a little fruit growing on a spiny cactus. He picked one, sliced it in two, and popped a half in his mouth and in his weakened state did his best to eat it. It was "of good taste." A moment later, the corporal began coughing up gobs of "fetid" blood. "He continued eating others," the priest wrote, "and each time he found himself better able to eat them." The corporal returned with fruit for his shipmates to try. They liked it so much they rowed back out to the island for a proper harvest. Their swollen gums returned to normal and their teeth became "tightened and fast." Just like that, they were cured.

The scientifically naive crew didn't know they had scurvy, a deficiency of vitamin C—they thought the illness was brought on by an ill wind. Nor did they know the mysterious little fruit contained large amounts of the very vitamin they lacked. All they knew is what they felt. The fruit tasted good, and after eating it the crew felt good.

During the California gold rush, outbreaks of scurvy killed

thousands. Bodies were dumped in the mountain snow or buried in makeshift graves. In winter of 1848–49, a miner named Edward Gould Buffum found himself, along with half of his camp, laid up with swollen legs and bleeding gums. He would have died if not for the accidental discovery of some beans growing next to a path. Buffum lived on them for a week, then dragged himself into town, where he spent $3 a pound for potatoes (about $100 per pound by today's value). The preferred preparation was to slice them raw and dress them in vinegar, a recipe whose peculiarity is exceeded by its nutritional potency. Raw potatoes have much more vitamin C than cooked ones, and the acid in vinegar protects vitamin C from breaking down. This strange but medicinally potent salad wasn't discovered by scientific research or recommended by doctors. It was born of craving. Some internal impulse drove these men to supply their bodies with what was so desperately needed.

During the era of slavery, American slaves experienced their own "depraved appetites," cravings so strong as to be considered "ungovernable." Their object of desire was not fruits and vegetables, however—it was earth. The cause, according the leading minds of the time, was the standard trifecta of moral failings: weakness of character, depravity, and a tendency toward vice. In 1833, a doctor named David Mason informed his peers they had it all wrong. Earth eating wasn't a disease but "actually a kind of remedy." The practice, he pointed out, was common all over the tropics—pregnant women in Indonesia, for example, would bake cakes out of clay and eat them. Why? Because earth contained "useful ingredients." Earth eaters, Mason noted, preferred a kind of clay tinged red by iron. The compulsion to eat earth, in other words, was caused by an iron deficiency. As a 2014 study recently put it, when it comes to earth eating, low blood iron is "a clear marker of risk."

Pellagra is nearly nonexistent today, but in 1989 there was a mass outbreak in the African country of Malawi at a camp for refugees fleeting a civil war in neighboring Mozamique. The refugees did indeed develop skin scales, as the textbooks would have you expect, but they were not the first symptom. "They complained about the lack of groundnuts," says Dr. Marc Gastellu Etchegorry, a French doctor who was the chief of mission for Doctors Without Borders in Malawi at the time. "Nuts are a usual part of diet in Mozambique," Dr. Gastellu Etchegorry says, "and they reminded us often." What they *wanted*, once again, was what they *needed*.

In cases of extreme nutritional need, "wanting" could reach such a severe intensity that to simply be awake was to be in pain. Grown men would have dreams of eating fruit only to wake up sobbing. The drive to eat earth among slaves was so powerful it was described as an "addiction" and an "invincible craving." To control it, slave owners, in their dependably inhumane and ghastly immorality, resorted to fitting slaves with iron masks.

When "wanting" finally acquired the desired goal, humans did not behave like snakes. We did not robotically swallow our food and then nap. We experienced gale-force levels of "liking."

In 1848, an Irish nationalist named John Mitchel was thrown aboard a British ship bound for a penal colony in Tasmania and developed scurvy during the Atlantic crossing. When the ship made port in Brazil, fresh provisions were brought on board that included freshly baked loaves of bread, which not only were rich in calories but would have tasted incomparably better than the stale ship's rations. But Mitchel avoided the bread. He chose instead to purchase a farcically large quantity of fresh oranges. "I became proprietor of thirty for sixpence," he wrote in his journal, "and shall never, never wish to forget the brutal rapture with which I devoured six of them on the spot." It was a banner day for the wisdom of the body. The oranges brought the vitamin-C-deficient Irish nationalist to a state he described as "brutal rapture." "Wanting" told Mitchel what he needed. And the fevered state of "liking" those oranges brought on told him that what he was eating was good.

The system worked. "Liking" may feel good, but it is, ultimately, a tool—one that lets us optimally exploit our surroundings. A snake has to settle for whatever winds up in its fanged maw. Humans, on the other hand, want the best, because the best most perfectly suits the requirements of living.

10

You Are Eating Pig Feed

I f the human appetite can be driven by specific needs, what happens if you stop that need from ever arising in the first place? For example, let's say you traveled back in time and dispensed vitamin C pills to the thousands of British seamen who were destined to fall ill with scurvy. Would you cure scurvy before it even started?

The answer is an easy yes. Thanks to their replete nutritional status, not only would the sailors have remained in good health, but their yearning for fruits and vegetables never would have awakened in the first place. They could have merrily sailed the ocean blue eating salt beef and hardtack without ever knowing the pain of swollen gums or pitching the bodies of their dead shipmates overboard. Vitamin C pills would have saved lives numbering in the millions.

What would happen if you did the same thing today? If everyone swallowed a vitamin C pill each morning, would this reduce our inclination to eat fruits and vegetables? If so, would these effects take place within days or would they not show up for decades? Would such a shift in eating be good or bad? Maybe if people stopped eating fruit, which has sugar in it (though not much), we would all lose a little weight. Then again, perhaps just the opposite would happen. With the inclination to eat fruits and vegetables satisfied by a pill, people might well eat more of the wrong things—more potato chips, hot dogs, ketchup, and sugary drinks. Then again, maybe nothing would happen at all.

An experiment very much like this one began in 1941, when the American government initiated its policy of encouraging the "enrichment" of refined flour with B vitamins, which would go on to effectively become law. Just like that, four micronutrients— niacin, thiamin, riboflavin, and iron (a mineral)—were turning up in everyday foods such as white bread, pie, cake, cereal, rice, and grits. For the first time in the history of our species, it was possible to get B vitamins in a food where they'd never before existed—refined carbs.

The policy wiped out pellagra. But were there side effects? As government policy instruments goes, the enrichment laws, it must be said, were blunt. Only a tiny subpopulation of Americans suffered from pellagra, but the cure—adding B vitamins to flour—applied to every living American, the vast majority of whom hadn't the slightest need for it. Did fortification—or "enrichment," as it is known if the government does it—affect them? Did all that niacin, thiamin, and riboflavin change the eating behavior of a nation?

One way to explore that question is to examine which foods provided Americans with niacin prior to enrichment. A sizable contribution came from beans, the very food Joseph Goldberger insisted on feeding to sick orphans. Prior to enrichment, the American bean story was a happy one. Bean consumption had steadily been ramping up and reached an all-time high in the early 1940s, at just under ten pounds per person per year. The future, you would think, should have looked rosy. The country was pulling itself out of the Great Depression and would soon enjoy the abundance and prosperity of the postwar years.

That's not how things turned out, however. As the nation's grain millers began adding B vitamins to refined flours, bean consumption began a long and dismal decline, finally bottoming out in 1980, just as the obesity epidemic was taking flight. Now that everyone was getting their niacin in bread, pasta, and doughnuts, it was as though the inner need for beans faded away.

Much stronger evidence that vitamins can and do affect both appetite and weight gain emerged just a few years after enrichment became law. The research was carried out at a facility in Urbana, Illinois, in the fall of 1947, and it would forever change the way much of the food we eat is produced. This research was not carried out on humans, however, but on pigs, which may explain why hardly anyone seems to have taken notice.

THE 1940s were heady times in pig farming. Thanks to the recent discovery of vitamins, pig farmers were on the cusp of realizing a long-held dream: raising their pigs on "drylot," a small fenced-off space where the animals eat, sleep, go to the bathroom, and even raise their young—what today is referred to as confinement.

The alternative to drylot was pasture, which sounds idyllic but to farmers brought a load of troubles. Out on pasture pigs would root and burrow, creating divots and ruts in fields that needed to be leveled if a farmer ever wanted to run a tractor over it. Every now and again, the neighbor's wife would knock on the door and announce her prized bed of carrots had just been destroyed. During summer pigs would get hot and dehydrated, and in winter they needed a warm place to bed down.

Things were so much easier on drylot. The pigs couldn't escape and they couldn't tear up fields. They hardly moved, and that was another bonus, because a sedentary pig converts more of its expensive food to valuable flesh.

The problem with drylot was keeping pigs properly fed. The richest feed of all was a mix of corn and soybeans. This blend was like rocket fuel—pigs gained weight and gained it fast. Even better, the feed was cheap and easy to store. But it had a huge drawback: if corn and soy was all you fed pigs, the pigs would eventually get diarrhea, their skin would turn yellow, they would vomit, lose all that valuable weight, their hair would fall out, and eventually they'd stop eating and start to walk funny. The diet, as one scientist dryly put it, was "inadequate for optimum growth." The pigs were suffering from a nutritional deficiency. And the cause, once again, was too much corn.

Out on pasture, however, where pigs could forage as they pleased, nutrition took care of itself. As the 1942 *Yearbook of Agriculture* put it, "Good pasture plants or a limited amount of well-cured roughage (particularly alfalfa), have proved to be of value as sources of essential nutrients." On pasture, the omnivore's dilemma of obtaining all the required nutrients was solved by all the different things there were to eat. Out in the field, pigs could indulge their omnivorous nature, and they did.

Vitamins changed everything. No sooner had these crystalline wonder substances been discovered than animal scientists started adding them to pig feed. Perfecting the formula took years of experimentation. The scientists would add a little of this vitamin along with a little of that, only to find the entire litter laid low with diarrhea.

Then came the experiment at the University of Illinois. The first group of pigs were fed a "basal ration" that was mainly ground corn and soybean meal. Though rich in carbohydrates and protein, it was, nevertheless, a nutritional disaster. The pigs' hair coat became rough, their skin flaked off, and they stumbled around in a slick of diarrhea. Though a mountain of feed made its way down their gullets, the pigs barely put on weight, only gaining a measly twenty-two pounds in sixty-five days.

The next group of pigs received the same corn-soy diet, only theirs included a sprinkling of the B vitamin riboflavin. The addition this single vitamin made was extraordinary. Weight gain nearly doubled from twenty-two to thirty-nine pounds, and it took the pigs a week less to gain that weight. Pantothenic acid, another B vitamin, boosted weight gain to forty-three pounds and shaved off another ten days.

When a blend of six B vitamins were added to the feed—riboflavin, niacin, pantothenic acid, thiamin, pyridoxine, and choline—the pigs experienced a superb uptick in what livestock professionals call feed efficiency. For the first group, it took 5.4 pounds of feed to gain a single pound of flesh. With each added vitamin, that number ticked down—3.5 pounds, 3.4, 3.1, and so forth. And when all the vitamins were added together, efficiency reached a stunning 2.9 pounds of feed per pound of weight gained.

Case closed. Vitamins make pigs gain weight.

Well, not so fast. A feed efficiency score of 2.9 might sound like a turbocharged rocket ship to obesity, but maybe those pigs only looked good because they were being compared to pigs dying of malnutrition. This experiment demonstrated that vitamins prevent nutritional deficiencies, but it did not show that vitamins can make pigs gain weight *faster*. And in animal science, that was the mission, because if your aim is to turn pigs into food, the faster and more efficiently a pig puts on weight, the cheaper its meat will be.

In 1954, the University of Illinois embarked upon another grand experiment. The object: to raise the fastest-growing pigs.

Effect of B Vitamin Supplementation on Weight Gain in Pigs

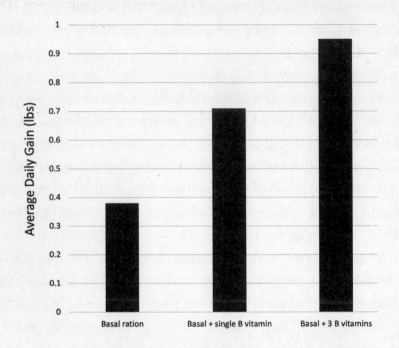

If this study were a reality show, it could well have been called *America's Biggest Gainer*.

There were four groups. Team A (my coinage) was fed a "mixed ration" created by an animal nutritionist that contained everything a pig needed—the corn, the soybean meal, meat scraps, dried whey—all fortified with vitamins. They lived on drylot. Team B also lived on drylot, but they were fed "free choice"—they got to choose between corn in one trough and a "supplement" in the other, which contained the vitamins, the protein, and everything else. Team C was like Team A—fed a mixed ration—but Team C was put on pasture, where they could also eat alfalfa and the like. And Team D was fed free choice, but also out on pasture. The scientists filled the feed troughs, then sat back and watched.

It was a blowout. Team A was the clear winner. The pigs that were fenced in on drylot and fed a mixed ration ate more, gained more, and had the thickest rind of white fat on their chops. The lesson was clear: if you wanted to get a pig fat, stick it in an enclosed space, and give it a nutritionally complete feed.

Animal science never looked back. In 1959, the University of Illinois produced a pamphlet titled "Balancing Swine Rations" which spread the new gospel of pig farming. "The pig," it said, "has a reasonable ability to balance his diet when fed on a free-choice basis." But that was old way. "Better results are possible today," it proclaimed with well-earned pride. Pigs "gain more rapidly when fed complete rations" and it was "no longer necessary to rely upon pasture as a source of vitamins and minerals."

Pigs were rousted off pasture and put on drylot and, later, into the "barns" they live in today, which are more like super-

Effect of Feed Type and Environment on Weight Gain in Pigs

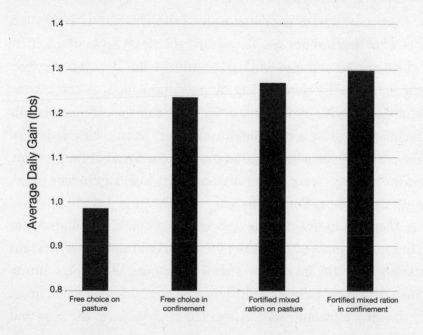

optimized flesh factories. Today, pigs can be fed up to four times as much niacin and twenty times as much riboflavin as in the 1950s, and they gain weight 40 percent faster. The mixed ration has reigned supreme for more than half a century.

But let's rewind the tape for a moment and watch the highlights in slow motion. Perhaps the pigs that came in last place—the ones that gained the least amount of weight—have a story we can learn from. That distinction went to Team D, the pigs on pasture that were fed "free choice." To paint the picture, these pigs were standing knee-deep in alfalfa with their high-energy corn feed in one trough and their "supplement" in the other. They were true slowpokes. They put on weight about 25 percent slower than the winners.

That, however, is all they were—slow weight gainers. There was nothing *wrong* with these pigs—their skin didn't turn yellow, there were no neurological impairments, no diarrhea. They represented what had been, just a few years earlier, the model of a healthy, vigorous American pig.

The most interesting detail about Team D is not what they ate, but what *they did not eat*. They didn't gobble down as much corn, which doesn't come as much of a surprise. But here is a surprise: these pigs barely touched the supplement, which, at first glance, seems to defy biology. Corn, as we know too well, is nutritionally incomplete on its own. Therefore Team D should have balanced the corn they ate with at least a moderate amount of supplement. So if those pigs were eating corn but very little supplement, how were they getting their vitamins?

There could only be one answer: the pasture. When given the choice between a scientifically formulated "supplement" and the alfalfa sprouting all around them, something in the pigs' brains said, *Alfalfa*.

It was as though mixing vitamins in with carbs flicked a switch inside the pigs. It made them eat differently. When given nutritionally complete feed, the pigs lost interest in greenery and became carb-munching, weight-gaining machines. But if the carbs were presented on their own—rich in calories but nutritionally incomplete—the pigs reverted to their omnivore ways. They foraged on alfalfa and dug up roots and did what pigs are born to do.

That was the true and lasting lesson of those experiments carried out in Urbana, Illinois, so many years ago. The difference between "normal" and "optimal" weight gain didn't come down to calories. It came down to vitamins. And it forever changed the way we raise livestock.

Is there a lesson for us humans? Yes. And the answer is that we are not slow-gaining Team D. We are Team A. Our processed carbs come prepackaged with the vitamins necessary to metabolize them. Weight gain is set to "optimal." It is the law. We eat like pigs and we gain like pigs.

DID I just say what I think I said? How could vitamins—which contain the word *vital*—possibly be bad? No doctor ever told a patient to cut back on the vitamins. The problem with processed foods, we are told over and over, isn't that they contain too much vitamins, but that they don't contain enough. Vitamins are pure and blameless. To even consider that vitamins could be implicated in obesity seems ignorant, like saying oxygen causes cancer.

But let's consider it.

A University of Toronto professor named Harvey Anderson was first struck several years ago by the thought that there might be some relationship between vitamins and obesity, when he observed that Americans were more obese than Canadians. As he began searching for differences between these two similar countries with similar food traditions, his attention was caught by vitamins. Americans consumed more of them. In both countries, the law mandated enrichment of refined carbs, but in the USA companies are permitted "discretionary" fortification of foods. They can legally add certain vitamins as they please, which makes the nutritional info panel appear "healthier." As a result, for decades the collective American vitamin dose has steadily increased. "There are vitamins in breakfast cereal," Anderson told me in his office one afternoon. "There are vitamins in vitaminwater, and then people take vitamin pills." The breakfast cereal Total, he pointed out, contains a concentrated vitamin dose unequaled by any natural food. "It has everything." Pregnant women, he noted, are told not only to eat right, but to take multivitamins, meaning they are exposed to unnaturally high doses.

Anderson began to wonder, Are these huge vitamin doses a good idea? To find out, he began a series of experiments in which he fed female rats ten times the regular load of vitamins. "Lo and behold," he told me, "they all got fat." Like so many human mothers, the rat moms not only put on weight during pregnancy, they didn't lose that weight after giving birth—unlike rat moms on the regular diet. Their pups, furthermore, seemed to be preordained for a lifetime of weight gain. "We have a video clip of one of those rats at around a year old," Anderson told me. "It's nearly one kilogram." (That is very large for a rat.)

This seeming paradox begins to make sense when you look at what vitamins—specifically the B vitamin family—actually do inside the body. Each plays its own highly specialized biochemical role. Thiamin, for example, "plays a central role in the release of energy from carbohydrates." Riboflavin "is involved in release of energy in the electron transport chain." Niacin plays "an important role in energy transfer reactions in the metabolism of glucose, fat, and alcohol."

One word is common to every description: *energy*. The human body uses B vitamins to convert the calories we eat into energy the body can use. They are essential to metabolizing calories the way spark plugs are essential to a gasoline engine. Without spark plugs, gasoline is useless. And without B vitamins, calories are useless.

That's what happened to the pigs in that "basal" group in 1947. They ate a mountain of calories in the form of corn, but barely gained weight because they lacked the vitamins necessary to make those calories usable. It was the same for poor Southerners at the turn of the last century. They ate an outrageously energy-dense diet: cornmeal, molasses, and pork fat. But without the right vitamins, all that energy was unusable and passed right through them. Without niacin, all those calories could not be used as fuel.

There is a lesson here. These energy-metabolizing chemicals are "necessary" for obesity. We consume more calories today than we used to—everyone knows that—but we also consume more of the vitamins necessary to metabolize them. In 1920, the average American consumed about 1.4 milligrams of thiamin each day, which is just over what scientists recommend an average male consume. Then the government set out on the path of "enrichment" and gave companies the green light to add vitamins themselves. Today the food supply isn't enriched with vitamins so much as drenched. A serving of Kellogg's Froot Loops Tropical—without any milk—has at least 20 percent of the daily requirement of five vitamins. That is a lot of calorie-metabolizing potential. The average American now takes in three milligrams of thiamin per day. It may sound minuscule, but this is the thiamin requirement for a 550-pound man. With great obesity comes great B vitamin intake.

It can seem sacrilegious to implicate these wonder chemicals in obesity, but that's all they are: chemicals. Chemicals are neither good nor bad, but they can act in ways that surprise us. Curt Richter, one of the great biologists of the twentieth century, found that when it came to eating, B vitamins could act like strings pulling the limbs of a puppet. "The ingestion of thiamin chloride," he wrote, "particularly stimulated the carbohydrate appetite." Riboflavin had a similar effect on the appetite for fat.

Of all the B vitamins we drizzle into the food supply, the most worthy of scrutiny is the one connected to pellagra: our old friend niacin. As far back as 1949, scientists at the National Institutes of Health discovered that among the many different carbohydrates—glucose, dextrin, maltose, sucrose, fructose, and so forth—two, and only two, had an unusual relationship with niacin. For rats to gain weight while consuming these two carbohydrates, they required at least three times as much niacin as compared to other carbohydrates. If they didn't get an extra-large dose of niacin, they would develop a deficiency. What were those two carbohydrates? Sucrose and fructose—the first we know as table sugar and the second is a component in high-fructose corn syrup. Put more simply, if you're going to eat a lot of sugar and metabolize that sugar, you need to eat a lot of niacin, too.

Well, we do eat a lot of sugar. The average American consumes 105 pounds of sugar and high fructose corn syrup annually, and it is widely believed that this is playing a direct role in obesity and poor health in general. So what about niacin? We eat more than triple the required amount—to say nothing of what is consumed through vitamin supplements, which can triple that amount yet again. Too much sugar is, unquestionably, a dumb nutritional move. Perhaps too much niacin is, too.

"No one ever thinks about this on a human level," says Fred Provenza, a behavioral ecologist and professor emeritus of wildlands studies at the Department of Wildland Resources at Utah State University. Provenza spent forty years researching the effects protein or minerals, or even plant toxins, had on eating behavior, and if his experiments had a running theme, it was this: the animals had a habit of surprising him. "There are always 'downstream' effects," Provenza says. What an animal has eaten, or hasn't eaten, influences what it eats later, and how much it eats. "But you can short-circuit the whole system to get animals fat, if that's your goal," he says. "The animal scientists figured out how to do that decades ago."

The parallels between humans and livestock are too striking to ignore. Back in the day, you had to wait for a chicken, pig, or cow to grow up to become fat and delicious. The young ones were lean and stringy, which is how young animals, including humans, are supposed to be. Then the livestock industry figured out how to achieve "optimal growth." Thanks to the thermonuclear combination of concentrated calories and concentrated vitamins, farm animals achieve a buttery layer of plumpness while still in the bloom of youth. People do, too.

OVER IN Italy, the vitamin situation couldn't be more different. A typical Italian consumes around a single milligram of thiamin per day—less than what Americans consumed in 1940. Italians consume half as much niacin and riboflavin as Americans do today. Italians look more like Team D. Their growth is "normal," whereas in America weight gain is "optimal."

Italians have access to some legendary sweets, not to mention bottled juice and soda. Could it be that one of the reasons they don't overindulge is that on some level the Italian brain understands it doesn't have the niacin to metabolize all that sugar? Perhaps the vitamin is acting like a leash on weight gain.

If it all seems hard to comprehend, consider combustion. If an oil refinery caught fire, one obvious way to contain the blaze would be to reduce the supply of fuel. But if every measure you took to restrict the fuel supply failed, there is another less obvious but equally effective strategy: reduce the oxygen. So it is with metabolism. The calories in food are just pieces of potential energy, and without the vitamins, they aren't useful.

But even this view—where we picture a precise quantity of vitamins entering the body and metabolizing a precise quantity of calories, causing a precise amount of fat to accumulate—still misses a big piece of the human food puzzle. Vitamins don't just passively show up in the stomach. They must be consumed. Eating is a *behavior*. For an omnivore, balancing a diet is something you have to go out and do—like those goats of Olympic National Park who seek out human urine. Being an omnivore takes effort, and perhaps that effort is more important than we understand.

For example, if an Italian woman is struck by a desire for *lardo* draped over crusty bread, the enjoyment that such a snack brings simply cannot last. Why? Because it is not nutritionally sustainable. If *lardo* and bread were all that woman ate, she would eventually descend into pellagra.

That's not what happens. The brain collects data about what's entering the mouth, monitors and predicts changes to the "internal state," and serves up the urge to stop eating and turn to something else—beans, for example, or meat, broccoli rabe, cheese or yogurt. It course corrects. An Italian woman has to eat as humans were designed—as an omnivore. There are costs to doing that. Other foods have to be obtained. They have to be prepared. It isn't impossible to become obese in Italy, but it's much harder to pull off. You have to eat a wider variety of foods, and you have to eat more of them.

Now imagine an American eating white bread with butter, or doughnuts, cake or crackers, or any other combination of processed carbs and fat. No matter how much of these foods this person eats, his or her brain will never detect a nutritional imbalance, thanks to government-mandated fortification. The appetite for some other food will never be wakened. Thanks to ancient government policy, Americans can consume vast amounts of calories without running out of the vitamins necessary to turn those calories into fat.

Fortification is the Walmart approach to nutrition. You get everything in one spot. It's cheap, it's fast, and it's easy. But an omnivore was not designed to eat that way.

The Italian way of eating—the "old road"—is like shopping in a small town. You have to visit lots of little shops to get everything you need. It takes longer and it's more expensive. But as each need is met, a little burst of deliciousness—of "liking"—comes with it. Call it the omnivore bonus. It is a better way of eating. Those nutrients all exert their own pull and deliver their own little moments of rapture. Eating is a never-ending journey, fueled by pleasure.

It sounds bizarre when you think about it. How could it possibly be healthy to "need" a vitamin? But in other fields of biology, this is the normal way of things. When bones aren't regularly stressed by the freight of exertion, they turn brittle and weak. Without exercise, muscles atrophy. Coddling is the help that hurts. It is the little doses of harm that make us flourish.

This is the sad story of the American palate. While European children are moved to eat olives, pâté, and R-rated cheeses, we struggle to graduate from chicken nuggets and microwave pizza. We aren't unsophisticated or stupid. We just don't need what the Europeans need. We have strangled our inner omnivore. Like pigs in a barn, we gorge on a nutritional completeness we were not designed for. Meanwhile, the brain circuit that dispenses actual enjoyment—the quality-control center that rewards our behavior—is as shriveled as an old raisin.

For all its high-flying technology, modern food has not advanced the behavior we call eating. It has turned us into something more like dumb farm animals.

PART V

The Brain-Changing Power of Good Food

11

The End of Craving

nja Hilbert is a professor of behavioral medicine at the University of Leipzig, where she treats some of Germany's most extreme cases of obesity and disordered eating. Three-quarters of her patients have a body mass index of at least 40 and about a quarter are at 50 or above—a five-foot-five-inch woman who weighs 306 pounds, for example. Besides suffering from obesity, her patients also have, on average, two of the following five conditions: heart disease, diabetes, sleep apnea, arterial hypertension, and dyslipidemia (excess fat in the blood). Thirty-seven percent have major depression, 17 percent have PTSD, 9 percent have a panic disorder, and 9 percent have an alcohol use disorder.

Many of Hilbert's patients have a binge-eating disorder, a condition that, perhaps more than any other, illustrates the power of an inflamed desire for food. Binge eaters are periodically seized by sudden bouts of extreme craving that drive bursts of voracious, uncontrolled consumption. "They feel the food has control over them," Hilbert says, "that they cannot resist it." They eat rapidly, they eat unambiguously large amounts, and they eat when they aren't physically hungry. In extreme cases, they eat when it's physically painful to do so.

Their enslavement to food is so strong it can warp what most people regard as basic tasks of living. Hilbert, for example, often has to help patients develop a route from their home to the train station that shields them from the siren call of tempting food. "They are not able to set a goal, plan accordingly, or evaluate the outcome," she says. To her patients, the decision whether to take the stairs or the elevator is like being offered a limousine ride to the airport versus crawling there on all fours with your luggage chained to your neck. Buying and eating highly processed food can be so deeply ingrained that her patients have difficulty even comprehending that such a behavior can be changed. Their brains don't function the way healthy brains function.

People with obesity literally think differently, and those differences go beyond how they think about food. In a "stop-signal task," patients are instructed to press a left button or a right button according to certain rules until they hear a sound indicating they should stop. It's not complicated. Most people press the buttons, hear the sound, and stop. Not Hilbert's patients. "Obese people have more difficulty with this," Hilbert says, "especially people with binge-eating disorder." They can't stop pressing buttons. They have trouble bringing their most basic responses under control.

Women with obesity, in particular, score differently on these types of tests, including "delay discounting tasks." When offered a smaller reward now or a bigger reward later, they are more likely to opt for the smaller but more immediate reward. If you think of the brain's pleasure system as assigning value to what is useful, for people with obesity the temptations of the moment are more heavily weighted. This is considered a "cognitive dysfunction." This behavior is observed in victims of stroke, brain trauma, and neurodegenerative diseases—and obesity. The greater a patient's mental difficulties, the harder it is to lose weight.

These effects are also "bidirectional." These mental tendencies not only cause obesity, they bring about "comorbidities," such as diabetes, high blood pressure, and inflammation, that inflict yet more damage on the brain, taking a further toll on executive function. It is, as Hilbert says, "a vicious cycle."

Hilbert's job is to disrupt that cycle. The odds she faces are terrible. About 95 percent of patients who enter obesity treatment, she acknowledges, have either returned to baseline five years later or have gained weight. Six percent of her patients don't make it to the first appointment and a fifth drop out before the first year is up. Of that latter group, 35 percent just stop showing up, 33 percent have family or health-related problems, 9 percent say they don't have the time, and 3 percent die. Hilbert's patients have "the wish" to lose weight, but many are simultaneously stubborn and unwilling. "They get angry," Hilbert says. "They get very frustrated and become very defensive." About one in five will end up getting some form of bariatric surgery, in which the size of their stomach is surgically reduced. "I don't expect miracles."

Yet, there is the odd miracle. Hilbert has had patients lose sixty-five pounds in less than two years and keep it off—but she insists that success should not be measured by mind-blowing weight loss. Not gaining weight, she points out, is its own form of weight loss. This is particularly true for people with binge-eating disorder, who are poised for a lifetime of weight gain, sometimes as much as twenty pounds in a single year. If Hilbert can intervene and stop or limit further weight gain, she can spare patients years of anguish and ill health. This is why her patients perform stop-signal tasks and carefully plan how to get home from work.

If they can lose even a small amount of weight or just stay physically active, she says, they can experience improvements in metabolism, mood, anxiety, and body image.

WHEN IT comes to her own eating, Hilbert is more of a "liker" than "wanter." One of her oldest and best food memories is of her grandmother's oatmeal. The oats, grown by her uncle, would be soaked overnight and cooked the next morning with raisins, nuts, honey, and milk. Her father loved an intense whole-grain sourdough bread, baked in a wood-fired oven, called *Schwarzbrot*— literally "black bread." Hilbert couldn't stand it. "It was sour, bitter, hard to chew, unpleasant," she says. But with time she came to love it, too, particularly with ham and butter.

The idea that the relationship between the pleasure of eating and disordered eating was misunderstood first occurred to Hilbert when she was doing her master's at the University of Nancy, in France. French food, she found, was its own graduate-level education. The variety and quality of French cheeses astounded her. She is still floored by the memory of a Christmas Eve dinner she had in Normandy, which began in the early evening with champagne and did not conclude till the early morning. There was salad, oysters, cheese, roast goose stuffed with chestnuts, and the traditional holiday cake called *bûche de Noël*. Each dish was paired with its own wine. In all, seven courses were served. "They even had ritualized courses between the courses," Hilbert remembers, such as cider sorbet, to refresh the palate and revive the appetite.

A few years later, Hilbert was working in Paris and treated her colleagues to a typically German meal, sauerkraut braised with sausages, smoked pork, and white wine. During the meal, one of her colleagues asked Hilbert what kind of wine she used to make the dish. Hilbert couldn't answer. "In Germany, nobody would think of using a special wine from a specific region," she says. As Hilbert shrank into her seat with embarrassment, the conversation turned to wine, specifically ranking which wines made the best sauerkraut.

Even a simple one-pot dish of sauerkraut and sausages, it seemed, was an opportunity to plot the maximum experience of deliciousness. The French, Hilbert observed, loved sophisticated foods served at expensive restaurants. But they also loved simple, rustic dishes that were, as she puts it, more rurally prepared. "It was as if the sensuality of eating was part of their personality," she says. To so many obesity researchers, the tendency to indulge, over and over, in the pleasures of food and alcohol is incontrovertible evidence of humanity's unrelenting and unhealthy appetite. Hilbert, however, started to see things differently.

Soon after the stretch in France, she began working with patients with bulimia, an eating disorder that is often blamed on the prevalence of the unreasonably thin, hyperbeautiful images of females that young women are subjected to. Paris is considered the world capital of fashion, and the French visual environment is as saturated with unrealistic standards of female beauty as any other. Yet, Hilbert observed that Frenchwomen were not particularly overcome with bulimia as a result. As Hilbert scientifically expresses it, "The normative slenderness ideal in the population was not so much different from the negative body image of people with bulimia nervosa." In other words, the elevated standard of beauty in France should have exerted some negative effect on eating, but it did not. The reason seemed to be the relationship the French had with food. They reveled in the pleasure of eating, while Hilbert's patients with bulimia fought a war against it. "There were not able to enjoy food at all."

Compared to bulimia, obesity posed a different and refreshing challenge. Whereas people with bulimia could be rigid and controlling, her patients with obesity were spontaneous, impulsive, and likable. "I loved the things they would say," Hilbert remembers. Their relationship with food, however pathological, could be endearing. One patient, she remembers, would binge eat gummy bears, arranging an entire bag of them by color while doing the ironing—the greens, the whites, the reds, and so on. "There was a ritualistic component," Hilbert says. "It was touching." More important, Hilbert learned firsthand that when people tried to forcefully control their relationship with food, they ended up becoming tormented by it. Food played such an outsize role in the emotional lives of her patients that for some researchers in a lab coat to expect them to just extinguish that relationship seemed not only unrealistic but cruel.

In 2003, Hilbert moved to St. Louis for eighteen months to work with Denise Wilfley, a renowned expert in binge-eating disorder at Washington University. Soon after arriving, Hilbert developed eating challenges of her own. The fruits and vegetables were bland, the yogurt was so sweet it tasted like dessert, and the portions in the cafeteria were comically huge. The tentacles of America's disordered eating even reached inside a clinic devoted to studying it. Some of Hilbert's colleagues had the irritating habit of eating while they worked. "They would come into a meeting with one of those soups where you pour hot water into a plastic container. Everyone could smell it," she remembers, still put off, years later, by the cloying aroma. "Why can't you just have a coffee?"

The bread and bagels were flavorless and seemed to go right through her. "I never felt full," she says. "I would eat them and be hungry." Muffins were just as bad. Her partner, Jochen, a tree surgeon, sent her a recipe for a simple, wholesome bread that called for mixing about a pound of spelt flour—spelt is an ancient variety of wheat—with a pound of buttermilk, along with some salt and baking powder. Hilbert baked a loaf and was transported. It was delicious. It tasted like bread. It left a lasting feeling of "deep satiety"—a sense of satisfaction and replenishment that continued long after a meal had concluded. "This is a concept my field doesn't yet fully understand," Hilbert says. "We need to do more research. We need to learn how to measure this."

Hilbert eats Jochen's bread for breakfast without fail, except when traveling. For a data-driven scientist, a leader in her field, breakfast broaches the spiritual. It is a period of "mindful sensory immersion that guides the rest of the day." She spreads butter on the spelt bread and eats it with jam she makes from fruit in her garden. And always with Jochen. You could say the meal is as much about their relationship as it is about the food. But it's also about maximizing enjoyment. The flow of pleasure is, as the scientists say, "bidirectional." The food makes the relationship better, but the relationship makes the food better.

Hilbert made me see something that I had not realized. "Liking" is also "bidirectional"—a two-way street. Eating better food causes more enjoyment. But the enjoyment of food correspondingly fuels the search for better food. Italians, Hilbert points out, spend time eating together. She can list the cultural predilections the travel writers all describe but never explain. Italians eat slowly. They eat with family. And they prize food of a high quality. Hilbert understands the behavior's significance as only a scientist can. "This decreases the probability of eating fast food, eating at the office, or eating in the car," she says.

Put more simply, "liking" can be used as a tool against "wanting." Now that we have an idea of how the system really works, Hilbert is finding the buttons that can change it. And the news seems almost too good to be true. The greatest malady presently afflicting humankind may have the greatest of all possible treatments: food so delicious as to be brain altering. This is why, during some sessions, Hilbert will dim the lights and hand a patient one of the finest, most delicious, most wonderful chocolates in all of Leipzig, then give the following instruction: "Eat it."

WHEN HILBERT treated the woman who binged on gummy bears, Hilbert knew she could not expect the woman to simply stop. "You can't just take it away. But maybe you can *replace* it," she told me with almost a twinkle in her eye. One day during therapy, Hilbert sat the woman down and gave her a single fine Belgian chocolate with a soft center called a praline. She asked the woman to close her eyes, put the praline in her mouth, and let the warmth of her body melt the chocolate and reveal its creamy beauty.

"It comes as a surprise to them that such a small amount of food can provide this intense experience," Hilbert says. Drawing on all the behavioral training she had acquired under Hilbert, the woman was instructed to plan a visit to a chocolate shop and to buy a single praline—just one. When she was seized by the craving for gummy bears, she was to eat the single praline and nothing else.

It worked. The flair of "wanting" was extinguished, as though dowsed by a shower of "liking." The expectation of quantity was violated by intense quality. It was a first-round KO.

Dark chocolate helped Mary, another of Hilbert's patients with binge-eating disorder. Mary grew up in a large, underprivileged family and had two older brothers who would get drunk and then sexually abuse her. The family would then soothe the traumatized little girl with food.

The binge eating started when she moved away from home. "There was no one around to watch me and judge me," she says, and the volcano of "wanting" finally erupted. During the day, Mary would sit and plan out magnificent shopping sprees. She would imagine chips, always cheese-and-onion flavored. At the grocery store, she visited each aisle like a bee pollinating a meadow. If she bumped into someone she knew, she would tell them she was having a dinner party. The eating sessions that followed would appear identical to a starvation response. Mary would eat and keep eating until her belly hurt. "Then I would wait until my belly did not hurt anymore," she said, "and start again."

The new cravings are different from the old ones. Brighter and less controlling, she says. Dark chocolate, she found, tasted bitter and intense at first, but over time it worked a kind of magic. Soon, milk chocolate began to taste too sweet. "You have to eat dark chocolate slowly," Mary points out. "You can't lose control with it." She has developed other new likes, too. She loves plain yogurt with fruit. The creamy, pointed sourness of the yogurt is quenched by the sweetness of the fruit. "I have relearned how good these foods are," she says. She likes kohlrabi so much she sometimes craves it. It is a slow process, but her craving for food is decreasing while her enjoyment of it expands.

The old cravings aren't completely gone. They come back, especially during periods of stress. But after six weeks of therapy with Anja Hilbert, of stop-signal tasks, a treatment called beta-wave therapy, and captivating morsels of dark chocolate, Mary is seven pounds lighter. She is also a different person. "I still get very excited about cake," she says, "but then I taste it and it's not as good as I hoped." She has learned the truth about "wanting," that it can whisper sweet lies but deliver nothing. Now Mary can see her craving for food for what it really is: a desire that will never be satisfied. The jig is up.

By thinking this way, by opening the door to enjoyment, to "liking," we now have a means of getting "wanting" under control. And the reason is as follows: "Wanting" is stubborn, powerful, and inflexible. It won't listen to most earnest pleadings to go away, as any dieter or drug addict knows. But it will listen to "liking." The two brain circuits talk to each other. They exchange information at a rate difficult to put in words. Scientists have seen this in action with brain-scanners. You can think of "liking" as the con-sigliere to "wanting"—the only confidant it trusts. "Liking" is the key that opens the door that's always been locked.

The implications are, literally, life changing. Deliciousness is by no means the cause of our eating problem. But it is part of the cure. A blast of concentrated "liking"—of "brutal rapture," as the Irish nationalist John Mitchel put it—can extinguish a roaring blaze of "wanting." It sounds too good to even be possible. But Anja Hilbert showed me that it is true.

THE SECOND-TO-LAST thing I did with Anja Hilbert was open a bag of chips. Cheese and onion, Mary's favorite. I was taking part in a "cue-exposure task." It is easy to speak and think abstractly of "wanting" and "liking." Anja Hilbert has developed therapies that distill each into its essence, and now I was about to experience them both.

"Chips are all about 'wanting,'" Hilbert explained. Before I'd even eaten them, they were sending my brain information, coaxing it into desire. There was the image of the chips on the packet, the pop sound the bag made as I opened it, and the whoosh of zesty aroma. Chips. The exercise was working. The technique was initially developed as a treatment for phobias. If a person is afraid of spiders, the thinking goes, expose them to spiders until spiders lose their fear-inducing effect. It was later found that it can have a similar effect on people under the irrational sway of food.

At six feet one and 170 pounds, I am one of the lucky few not fighting a losing war with food. I do not meet a single one of the clinical criteria for binge-eating disorder. But Mary and I are not so different, at least not always.

If I walk into a party and there is a bowl of chips, I become aware of it. I mentally begin tracking it. Dopamine. The "getting stuff" system is revved into action. I could play Ping-Pong or get pulled into conversation, but the chips will be there at the edge of my awareness, an old friend calling out to me. When I eat them, I find myself grabbing the largest handful possible. My mouth sometimes feels too small. Disgusted, I wash my hands and mentally move on. Then I relapse and eat more chips.

If someone asked me to create a list of my hundred favorite foods, chips would not be on it. I can mentally relive eating certain steaks, I can rank the best cheeses and recall certain wines, standout peaches, mushrooms, burgers, sausages, sashimi, a wild snow goose a friend of my father's shot. My mother's cherry pie. But if you asked me point-blank, "Do you want some chips?" I would reach out my hand without considering it. If you offered me two plates, one with chips and the other with, say, a piece of Stilton on a cream cracker, my hand—my idiot hand—might actually go for the chips.

"Chips are pure 'wanting,'" Hilbert said.

She now set about to coaxing that "wanting" to its peak. "Feel the chips. Smell them," she urged like the emperor in *Star Wars* coaxing me to the dark side. She let me take a bite, but only a tiny one, "just so you get the taste." Crunch. Fade. Then she said "rub the chips together." It struck me as a silly thing to do. The sound was quiet, like sandpaper on soft wood, but it unblocked some inner dam. My desire for the chips shot to level ten. It was starting to hurt.

Kent Berridge, the neuroscientist and scholar of pleasure, has written about this, how "wanting" has a short temper. When it is severed from "liking," he writes, it becomes a "counterfeit pleasure" and can flip into anxiety, frustration, and fear. This insight is as modern as it is ancient. The word *tantalize*, Berridge points out, comes from a Greek myth about a wicked king named Tantalus, who is condemned by Zeus to spend eternity beneath the branches of a tree whose fruit he can never grasp while standing in a pool whose water he can never drink. "Wanting" only feels good if you believe "liking" is within reach. Otherwise, it's torture.

So many of us are like that strange Greek figure, caught in that endless loop. Each bite just fast-forwards us to the anticipation of the next bite. We confuse this sham pleasure for the real thing. And when we try to break free of "wanting," we just fall for another of its charms. What is dieting, after all, but yet another desire, a promise of deliverance that has almost no hope of coming true.

* * *

I NEVER did eat those chips. Hilbert instructed me to repeat the cue-exposure task with a fresher, crisper pair of chips. Once again, I inhaled the savory zing. I rubbed them together. Craving rushed in like a wave that crested and held until the pain of not eating became unbearable. But then, slowly, it began to recede. Like the calm that descends after a torrential storm, "wanting" began to fade. In time, the chips weren't chips anymore. Just two slices of industrially fried potato covered in chemical seasonings staring back at me. I stood up and threw the full, uneaten bag of chips in the garbage.

Now it was time to experience firsthand the object of the never-ending quest. It was time to experience "liking" at its purest. It was time to violate expectations.

"This exercise," Hilbert said, "was developed to show how much pleasure there is in one piece of chocolate." She dimmed the lights and directed me to place inside my mouth a square of dark chocolate with little pointed edges surrounding a crispy biscuit center. "You can close your eyes if you like." I did.

There was no pleasure to speak of, at first. The chocolate sat there like a child sulking in the corner. Then the melting began. Just a hint, then a droplet of liquid chocolate landed on my tongue. The drip became a trickle, then a rivulet that pooled. There was a plume of chocolatiness. It was not overwhelming, more like a cashmere blanket of cocoaness. I pressed the chocolate against the roof of my mouth with my tongue, and it left a luxurious smear.

Hilbert said something, but it didn't register. I had entered the realm. Just as the chips sped eating up, the chocolate was slowing everything down. A corner of biscuit poked through the chocolate coating. The biscuit. I had totally forgotten. *It is ruined*, I thought, turned to mush by saliva, but I maneuvered it between two molars, and it gave a satisfying crunch. I swallowed.

It's over, I thought. I sat there, grateful, but still in a state of "wanting." That magnificent chocolate was gone. I had guilty thoughts of seconds. But the thoughts were interrupted because the chocolate, I realized, was not gone. Its flavor lingered, like the slow fade-out of a song. This is what fancy wine types call the finish. I listened. I basked in its nuances until I found, to my surprise, that desire had been quenched. I was satisfied.

I opened my eyes. Hilbert was sitting at her desk, like some shaman who'd just taken me to the edge of the universe and back. We both smiled.

12

Can This Be Fixed?

So here, then, is the theory spelled out: the obesity epidemic is being fueled by advancements in food technology that have disrupted the brain's ability to sense nutrients, altered eating behavior, and given food an unnatural energetic potency. This is not an all-encompassing theory that claims to explain each and every instance of overweight or obesity. But this is *the* change. This is what set so many of us on a path to weight gain. We changed food and it changed us.

Humans are animals. We have big brains, small stomachs, and speedy metabolisms. We evolved in an environment where we needed to acquire the big macronutrients along with the multitude of tiny micronutrients. And we had to get it—all of it—efficiently. "Wanting" draws us to what we need. The nose and mouth sense information about food, and the brain processes the data. And "liking" delivers an instant, actionable report. It is nutritional computation that is *felt*.

For hundreds of millions of years, every one of our ancestors labored to feed themselves. Some won, some lost. But when food was obtained, it didn't tell lies. Fat tasted like fat. Sugar tasted sweet. And only strawberries tasted like strawberries. Food may have been scarce, but once you got hold of it, the game was over. The better it tasted, the more useful it was. When it came to eating, the quest for pleasure was the quest for nourishment. It worked.

Then, in a blink of a few decades, we changed food. So much of what we now eat is engineered to mislead the brain. The information we sense as we eat has become unreliable. We react as any animal reacts to uncertainty—by cranking up motivation. We avoid losses and seek the certainty of calories. It is the most significant change in food since the dawn of agriculture.

If that were not bad enough, we have used our limited nutritional knowledge to dumb down our omnivorous nature. Not long ago, achieving nutritional completeness required a kind of inner genius. That's why we created recipes and ate strange plants and animal organs and sometimes dirt. Now eating has become an easy, boring holiday. We are like pigs at the trough. Calories are everywhere. They come packaged with the vitamins necessary to turn those calories into fat. It is a perfect storm for weight gain.

So FIRST, the good news. If you are one of the 0.7 percent of the people in the world who call Italy home, keep doing what you're doing. Stay on the old road. Treat yourself to a *gran fritto* and do not under any circumstance let the joy of eating be stained by the fear of carbs or fat.

Now for the bad news: you probably are not Italian. Chances are you live in a food environment in which bite after bite has been perversely engineered to promote optimal weight gain. All of which brings up an urgent question: How do we stop this? Every effort to curb weight gain has failed. We seem powerless to resist "wanting." What do we do?

We could fix the food environment. Denmark introduced a tax on foods that are high in saturated fat as a means of discouraging their consumption. Berkeley, Philadelphia, Seattle, and Boulder have implemented soda taxes. Hungary taxes food with unhealthy levels of sugar, salt, and caffeine. Mexico taxes "nonessential" foods with more than 275 calories per hundred grams.

So why not go whole hog? Ban everything in the food system that is unhealthy. Make all those additives that require a graduate degree in food science to pronounce illegal. Pass a bill that decrees that henceforth ice cream shall actually be ice cream. Force the food companies to sell authentic food and not some engineered facsimile.

And can we rethink the now-ancient practice of enriching processed carbs? It has been nearly a century since pellagra was wiped out. Are we still running dangerously low on niacin, riboflavin, and thiamin?* Some countries—wealthy, advanced, science-forward nations that include Denmark, Finland, France, Japan, Korea, Spain, and Sweden (and Italy, obviously)—do not fortify their flour with vitamins. Amazingly, they do not face epidemics of pellagra every spring. They do, however, have lower rates of adult and child obesity. Can consenting adults of voting age at least have the *option* of buying unenriched flour with their groceries?

So do it. Purge the food environment of the ingredients and additives that are setting our brains astray. If we can force companies to put airbags in cars and make people wear seat belts and

---

* Not all B-vitamin fortification is, by its nature, suspect. There is strong evidence that the addition of folic acid to the food supply prevents birth defects.

pay taxes, mow their lawns and obey traffic lights, is improving the quality of food we put inside our bodies such a ridiculous thought?

It is not. If we don't undo the damage we have wrought upon food, the disorder of inflamed hunger will only continue to gain strength. Consider, for a moment, just how amazingly bad things have gotten in such a short time. We look at snapshots of ordinary people in the 1960s or 1970s doing ordinary things—at the supermarket checkout, at outdoor concerts, sunning themselves at the beach—and sit stunned that at one time the default body type was skinny. If we don't stop this problem, it is sure to get worse. We can either do something or we can continue eating ourselves to death. Could the solution be any more obvious?

And that, right there, is the problem. Because as fixes go, the "fix what's wrong with food" approach is so intuitively correct that it obscures a deeper but more profound truth. This is yet another "do it by force" approach. By this point, it ought to have a familiar ring to it, and perhaps not a good one. It presumes, once again, that we know what needs fixing, and all we need to do is fix it. It presumes we can control human behavior the way a pilot controls a plane. This approach has a dismal track record. Every time we try to change the food system by force, there is an unexpected consequence. It started in 1941 with vitamins, and it keeps happening. We keep trying to muscle the food system to suit our needs. If it hasn't worked before, why would it work this time?

Like any solution, this one bears thinking through. For one thing, it will be a bitter fight. To tell people they can't eat something is to limit their freedom. Consider the money at play. The lobbyists. The quarterly dividends. The multibillion-dollar PR pushback. Consider the political controversy around something as simple as a soda tax, and ask yourself, how likely it is that the obesity epidemic can be wiped out by politicians? Consider the factions in the nutrition wars and the never-ending disagreements about what constitutes bad food, and ask yourself, How likely is it that we can even agree on a solution? Consider that over the last four decades, the collective effort to lose weight has achieved the opposite result: we have gained weight.

This isn't even a new idea. Every sane examination of our dysfunctional relationship with eating comes to the same conclusion: we need to eat "real food" instead of chemically engineered confections. We have called out junk food for what it is—junk—for decades. Yet we keep eating it and we keep getting heavier.

When you get right down to it, the desire to go out and fix the food system is just that: a desire. It is yet another expression of the disease itself. We already know it won't work. Because every time we have embraced some simple fix—whether it's a diet, the demonization of carbs or fat, or some idiotic form of coffee—it hasn't worked. It's easy to imagine a world where the food is pure and everyone is skinny and healthy again. But that's a wish. That is "wanting." The problem runs so deep it warps our ability to understand it.

Now consider this: Italians didn't do it by force. They never declared war on artificial sweeteners or fat replacers or passed a law that says, "All Italians must eat in the Italian way." Their food decisions come from the gut. They eat the way they eat for a simple reason: they *enjoy* it.

So as much as we need to change what's been done to food, we need to do something even more fundamental: change ourselves. We are expert "wanters." We have spent decades engaged in pseudoscientific discussions about food's abstract qualities—

fat, carbs, calories, vitamins—and we have ignored the only thing the brain truly cares about: actually eating it. Anja Hilbert doesn't treat obesity and binge eating by changing Germany. She treats it by changing her patients. We need to do what she does. We need to awaken that other neural pleasure circuit.

That, when you think about it, seems like the tallest order of all. If we cannot even change how much we eat, can we expect to go even deeper and alter the very functioning of our brains? Where do you even begin to look for an answer?

13

A Visit to the Old Road

Listen, listen to me, and eat what is good,
and you will delight in the richest of fare.

—ISAIAH 55:2

A word of advice: should you find yourself inside an elevator in Italy, treat the door-close button with respect. I pressed it repeatedly one morning just as my wife was stepping on. There were two results. The first is that my wife was bodychecked by a stainless steel Italian elevator door before her first sip of coffee. The second is that any elevated level of motivation, of "wanting," I harbored toward that door-close button evaporated. From then on, I pressed it only when needed, and I would only press it once.

I had come to Italy to answer a question. Why did Italy turn out so differently from America? After the discovery of vitamins, the road of nutrition forked. Governments faced with an epidemic of malnutrition could take the new road, as America did, and biochemically fix the problem, which seems like the obvious thing to do. Or they could stay on the old road.

Italy stayed on the old road. They could have fortified their flour but did not. They could have loaded their ice cream with alginate and other stabilizers and fats, but instead gelato shops boast their gelato is made in the artisanal, time-tested manner. It would be so easy to lower the counts on calorie bombs such as tortellini or mortadella with Simplesse and Avicel, but Italy sticks to tradition with pride. It is not because Italy is backward or economically underdeveloped. The north of Italy is a hot zone of wealth and industry. Yet its relationship with food couldn't be more different from America's. I wanted to know, once and for all, beyond the statistics, Why are Italians the way they are?

My attempt to find answers brought me inside a room in a building that was built in 1391 that is now part of Bologna's chamber of commerce. I was talking food with two women: Mariangela Venturi, who works for the chamber, and Alice Brignani, who is from the local tourist office. Mariangela had just retrieved the golden noodle. I imagined it would be kept behind glass, like a priceless artifact, but it spends its days inside a wooden box that looks like a tiny coffin. Mariangela removed the lid and set it on a table. The noodle is precisely eight millimeters wide, Mariangela said, and the length is 1/12,270th the height of the nearby Asinelli Tower, which sounds more significant than it is. We gazed at it for a silent moment, as though beholding some geometric truth.

"What happens if someone makes a noodle with the wrong measurements?" I asked.

"Nothing," Mariangela said.

The noodle was entered into the "depository" in 1972, yet somehow the recipe for the sauce—the *ragù*—didn't make it in for another ten years. This decade-long gap may have been the result of controversy, because the only thing more popular than food in Bologna is disagreement over how food ought to be prepared. Mariangela, for example, uses the official recipe when she makes *ragù*, but her mother does not. Alice doesn't use the official recipe either—her version doesn't include milk, but Alice hails from a family of *ragù* radicals. Her father's version substitutes sausage for pancetta. "There is no wrong way," Mariangela said.

But that's not true either, because Mariangela then shared the story of a Dutch TV crew that showed up in Bologna a year or so earlier with a slew of Dutch food products that bore the word *bolognese* on the packaging. Actual residents of Bologna were then given these products to taste, and their incredulous, hilarious responses were captured on video. "Everyone thought they were terrible," she said.

Mariangela eats pasta every day. Alice eats it every second day, but she works with a woman who eats pasta every day and never does any exercise.

"Is she . . . large?" I asked.

"No, she is okay," Alice said.

"Do people here ever go on diets?"

"We don't have obesity like you have," Mariangela snapped. "The way we eat is healthier." It was hard to argue with the keeper of the golden noodle. I had not yet seen, and would not see, a single person with obesity in all of Bologna. Every time a promising candidate loomed into view, it would end up being a tourist.

"Do you eat a lot of vegetables?"

"Of course!" Mariangela said. "As a side dish for the second course."

One such dish is *finocchi bolognese*, which is prepared by cutting a cooked bulb of fennel in half, scooping out the middle, and filling it with ground meat. You then dredge it flour, dip it in beaten eggs, coat it in bread crumbs, smother it in grated Parmesan cheese and butter, and bake it in the oven.

Rich food. Perhaps that was Bologna's secret, I thought. Anyone who can put away a plate of *finocchi bolognese* doesn't need to eat again until the summer solstice. There is no better recipe for everlasting hunger than eating light.

But then I realized I was seeing Italy through a foreigner's eyes. The foreigner sees what the foreigner wants, what the foreigner expected to see before the plane even landed—the pasta, the pizza, the lasagna. The foreigner won't touch the tripe (cow stomach) and never stops to think that headcheese and bitter chicory are every bit as Italian, and every bit as loved, as the lasagna. The tourists that flood Italy are intentionally clueless about all its regional peculiarities. I was determined not to be that kind of tourist. I wanted to know about the foods that made Italy, well, *Italian*. To understand the old road, you have to travel the old road.

A HUNDRED and thirty miles north of Bologna, tucked in the Dolomite mountains, sits the village of Lamon. Like every Italian city, village, and town, Lamon holds an outdoor food festival. It takes place in September and celebrates beans. It isn't listed in a single tourism brochure. No one I'd met thus far on my journey had even heard of Lamon except the chef at an extraordinary restaurant I visited in Veneto called Al Palazzino, who sources her beans there, along with whatever else grows in Lamon, because she believes the land to be special. Beans are interesting for another reason: Italians love them and Americans typically do not.

Enzo is a bean farmer, tall and lean with a handlebar mustache. At the annual bean festival, he was standing at a table covered in a checkered tablecloth, on top of which were packages of dried beans, a bowl filled with dried beans, and a digital scale. Enzo feels about beans the way people from Bologna feel about tortellini. He eats them for breakfast. When they're in season, he eats them every day, without fail.

Enzo is just average. Giuliano, trim and wearing a green V-neck, one-upped Enzo and announced that he doesn't just eat beans every day during harvest, but every day of every week, fifty-two weeks a year. He brews big pots of minestrone and depletes it, bowl by bowl. The flavor improves every day, he explained to me, until the pot runs dry and the cycle begins anew.

Exactly how one should prepare a Lamon bean is a matter of sometimes heated disagreement. Enzo celebrates a purism that verges on the severe: he boils his beans and then dresses them in a neutral vegetable oil. "I don't want the flavor of olive oil covering them up," he told me. An older woman named Margherita butted in to say that raw onion should be added during boiling. She was interrupted by another woman, who said, "Add rosemary, too."

These disputes are petty compared with the larger question of exactly which Lamon bean variety is the best. There are four: spagnol, spagnolet, canalino, and calonega. To anyone not from Lamon, they can be hard to tell apart. Locally, each bean has a devout following. According to Margherita, calonega is the best—unquestionably—because it has the thinnest skin. Tiziana, president of the consortium of bean growers, politely but strongly disagreed, saying spagnolet is the best.

This is when the thunderbolt struck. Here I was in an Italian mountain village, listening to yet another disagreement about food. No matter where I went or whom I talked to, all conversations about food invariably descended into disagreement. Even in the country with the most delicious food in the world, in a town famous for its beans, no one could seem to agree on anything.

There was, however, a difference. When Americans argue

about food, they bicker about nutrition. Carbs. Fat. Ketones. In-sulin. The glycemic index. Over in Italy, the quarrel is over reci-pes. Pancetta versus sausage. Spagnol or calonega.

It is the difference, I realized, between the old road and the new road. When pellagra raged, America blamed food. More than a century later, it still sees food as a slow-acting poison. In Italy, food wasn't the cause of pellagra—it was the solution. De-cades later, food's goodness isn't questioned so much as revered.

This is the quintessential American question about food:

How will this affect my body?

This is the quintessential Italian question about food:

Is this the best recipe?

For example, there is a major divide over polenta that has noth-ing at all to do with nutrition. Luciano Moro was raised on white polenta, which comes from white corn. According to his mother and father, yellow corn was what you fed pigs. When Moro was fifteen, he was visiting a friend when the friend's mother pre-sented him with a bowl of yellow polenta. Moro thought it was a prank. It was like someone placing a bowl of dog food in front of you. He thought the room would erupt in laughter, but quickly realized the situation was all too serious, and that his hosts, whose hospitality he had gladly accepted, fully expected him to not only put the yellow polenta in his mouth but to swallow it. Which he did. And it was good.

That any northern Italian even touches polenta is surprising, considering how many people died from eating it. Polenta is undergoing a revival, and Luciano Moro is leading the way forward, which is to say backward.

Moro won't touch supermarket polenta. Neither will his aunt, Rita Moro, who explained its two essential flaws. The first is that it's made from modern hybrid corn, the vast majority of which is grown as feed for animals—it really is pig feed. The second is that the germ is removed during milling, which lengthens the shelf life and speeds up the cooking, but at the cost of flavor. Real polenta is more expensive, and you have to store it in the freezer so the oils didn't go rancid. But when you eat it, the flavor makes it all worth it.

One of Luciano Moro's favorite varieties is called *badoera*, which once covered untold acres of Italian countryside but had all but vanished by the middle of the last century, thanks to the advent of ultraproductive hybrid corn. A few years ago, a businessman Moro knew was on vacation in Brazil when he came across a familiar-looking white corn and smuggled seeds back to Italy by hiding them among his rosary beads. It was *badoera*. Today Moro grows it and mills it along with eleven other rare varieties. Another is called *dente di cavallo bianco*, which means "horse tooth white." It is sweet and goes well with fish, Moro says. He talks of corn varieties almost as though they were his children—filled with potential, in need of protection and nourishment, and objects of unconditional love. At a local restaurant, we tasted a variety called *russo San Martino*, which appeared in a classic peasant dish with beans and radicchio, which sounds like a form of vegan torture but is very good. Bologna was two hours away by car, but a world away culinarily speaking.

Rita Moro lives on the farm where she grew up, which sits at the end of a long and thin winding road in backwoods Veneto. At seventy-six, she still raises chickens, geese, tomatoes, pumpkins, and corn. She learned to cook from her mother, who grew up eating polenta and beans every night and polenta with milk every morning. On weekends, the family would have polenta with broth or, if they were lucky, polenta with chicken. A single chicken was shared between thirty-five people, and the men who worked the field always got a bigger piece. Life was good. Her family owned their farm, which meant they ate every day. Other families did not. By the time Rita was born, in 1942, pellagra was gone but the stigma remained. "If you wanted to offend someone," she said, "you'd say they were a *pellagroso*—full of pellagra." No one says that anymore. But in the winter, it might as well be 1948 at the Moro farm, because Rita eats polenta and beans almost every evening. "It's the best dish we have."

Rita brought out an old, huge black pot from the kitchen. It was filled, as it had been so many times, with steaming white *badoera*. She spooned some onto a plate for me, then handed me a hunk of Montasio cheese. Polenta and cheese is nearly as classic as polenta and beans. Everyone began eating and, a moment later, commenting on the polenta. Christina, one of many family members who showed up to take part in the meal, said, "The supermarket polenta tastes like chicken feed."

"This tastes more like polenta," Rita said.

Lard is another thing that's changed since the old days. So many people have switched to olive oil you can hardly find lard anymore. I asked Rita why. "Because no one works the fields anymore," she said. "The appetite changes as the work changes."

She sounded like Michel Cabanac. The appetite in tune with bodily need. But Rita's point was bigger than that. The whole world thinks Italians still eat a "traditional" diet, which simply is not true. They eat more meat, more cheese, more olive oil, less lard, less wine, and less pasta (but still a lot of pasta). Yet, some-how, the nation's collective weight hadn't ballooned.

We often try to characterize the Italians, especially when it comes to food, by all the things they don't do. They don't drink a lot of soft drinks. They don't eat in the car or in front of the TV. They don't eat a lot of fast food. They don't eat microwave pizza. They don't drown their pizza in melted cheese.

Of all the words to describe Italian eating, *don't* is probably the worst. All the negatives in the world will never add up to a pos-itive. And the Italian relationship with food is a raging positive.

The secret, I think, comes down to something a chef back in Bologna named Pino Mastrangelo said to me. We were seated at a restaurant called Gigina, whose recipe for *ragù* has not changed since it opened in 1956, and where Mastrangelo was the chef up until a few years ago, when he joined a restaurant in Los Angeles called Uovo. (Pasta is handmade in Bologna and flown overnight to California.) We had had just put away a feast that included mortadella, steak tartare, tortellini, tagliatelle in *ragù*, and a fried veal cutlet filled with ham, cheese, and, to really take things to the limit, white truffle, when I began pelting him with questions. Why are Italians always arguing about recipes? Why don't they fortify their flour? How do they remain skinny amid such excellent food?

Mastrangelo sat for a moment and thought. "It comes down to the difference between feeding and eating," he said. "Italians don't want just to feed themselves, they want to *eat*." He paused again. "They want an *experience*."

EXPERIENCE. IT was the perfect word. Yet, why was this word so rare? The behaviorists didn't believe experience was real. Sci-entists still render the carnal act of eating into lifeless abstraction with words like *motivation*, *intake*, and *reward*. Can a science bleached of human experience ever hope to understand it?

In all the research I had conducted—the interviews, the conferences, the books, journal articles numbering in the hundreds—this word, *experience*, would show up in only one place, and always in connection to a single person. A person who also traveled to Italy to eat extraordinary food. That person was Johann von Goethe. Not only did this man conduct his life as though striving to capture and describe every experience and pleasure, his most famous literary work tells the story of a man who sells his soul to the devil not so that he can experience life at its best, but at its most intense.

This unceasing quest to experience made Goethe a great artist and a great statesman. Most amazing of all, it also made him a great scientist. This incomprehensibly talented individual—a man whose life achievements include running a small country, writing one of the world's great works of literature, and inspiring a generation of men to wear custard-yellow pants—was also one of the most original scientists of his era. He invented a weather-predicting device known as the Goethe barometer. His fascination with geology fueled a rock collection that numbered 17,800 samples. He wrote an influential work on the structure of plants as well as a book on the theory of color. His least known accomplishment may be his most impressive: Goethe discovered the cause of pellagra. More than a century before Joseph Goldberger visited that orphanage in Mississippi, Goethe pinpointed the disease's origin. In his diary entry dated September 14, 1786, he wrote, almost offhandedly, as though it were as obvious as the sun, that the cause of the peasants' malady was their high-corn diet.

So if we think "experience" has something to tell us about the puzzle that is food and eating, perhaps Mr. Goethe has something to tell us. What is it that he saw in the world that we don't?

Goethe, simply, saw life. But he saw it in a way to which his contemporaries were blind. The scientists of his day understood animals as biological machines. Like clocks or windmills, animals were driven by complex internal mechanisms, with muscles and organs in place of gears and springs. What distinguished one animal from another was its parts—this bird has a distinctive beak, that lizard has long claws, and so forth. For Goethe, that was the problem. Scientists could see what made animals different from one another, but they could not see what unified them—what made living things different from dead things.

Living things, Goethe believed, were different from nonliving things in two fundamental but important ways. First, living beings were pervaded by "wholeness." An ordinary leaf, for example, is a tiny version of the plant on which it grows. It contains the same cells, the same circulatory system, and the same fuel (sugar). The form of the leaf, furthermore, repeats itself all over the plant throughout its life, from the tiny leaves you find in an unsprouted seed, to the flower petals that ultimately create the next generation of plant. "From top to bottom," Goethe said, "a plant is all leaf.

The force of gravity, we now know, contains a similar wholeness. Gravity was long thought of as a force that draws objects in, but physics has turned that thinking on its head. Big objects don't attract smaller ones, the way a vacuum cleaner sucks in dirt. Gravity, rather, is the effect that every other piece of matter in the universe has on a particular object. It can seem difficult to comprehend, but Einstein imagined it thus: If there were only one particle in the universe, it would have no gravity. It would float about, weightless and attracted to nothing. But as soon as another particle is added, even just a speck of dust, each particle imparts some tiny amount of gravity to the other. In that sense, gravity is like a reflection of the entire cosmos in a single object. The whole visible in the part.

Machines are nothing like that. Machines are dead, and their parts, which also are dead, tell you nothing about the whole. The windshield wiper from a 2012 Honda Accord reveals nothing about the car it came from. You could x-ray it, dissolve it in acid, peer at it through a microscope, but you still wouldn't know anything about the steering wheel, the upholstery, or the stereo—or that it even came from a car in the first place. With machines, the part reveals nothing about the whole.

Machines, furthermore, run on fuel—pure energy. Living beings require more than that. Eating is not refueling. Eating is an effort to maintain wholeness. "Wanting," in that sense, is like gravity—a reflection. If there were only one object in the universe and that object was a ripe peach, it would not be delicious. But if you add another object to that universe—a person—deliciousness springs into existence.

The second quality Goethe saw in living beings was even grander: *design*. The natural world was filled with designs that recurred over and over. A bone that was part of a paw in one animal was, clearly, part of a fin in another, formed a hoof in another, and a hand in another. To Goethe, a skeleton wasn't just an organism's bones, it was a biological blueprint. These designs, furthermore, weren't static and unchanging. The design of a creature changed as it moved through life. Each species, furthermore, was like a snapshot of a particular instance of a grander, deeper plan.

Goethe called this the "the doctrine of metamorphosis" and considered it "the key to all signs of nature." Do not let the grandiose seventeenth-century language intimidate you. It means, at its simplest, that living things change in a way that dead things do not. A computer, which is a machine, works until one day it stops working. There is no journey, no arc of existence. It is not born, and it does not bloom into the fullness of life, reproduce, and then die. It does not seek gains and avoid losses. It just stops working one day.

Living things change and do not stop changing from the moment of conception. A girl who has just eaten an apple is, by comparison, a tick closer to becoming a woman than before she ate the apple. A leopard that drags a dead gazelle up a tree not only replenishes itself and grows, it is one step further from birth and one step closer to death. Evolution is, at the most elemental level, a story of change. Living things are like rivers—never exactly the same twice. We are always in flux.

AS WITH pellagra, Goethe was light-years beyond his contemporaries. Darwin would call him an "extreme partisan" of the theory of evolution. Goethe's understanding that in living things the part expresses the whole prefigured the discovery of DNA by nearly two hundred years.

If Goethe could step into our time, what would he say about food? I don't believe he would think much of the Hungry Ape Theory. He would tell you that figs taste far too good for the measly payload of calories they carry. He would point out that the deepest study of nutrition and physiology, in all its molecular intricacy, tells you nothing about eating. A thousand PhDs' worth of research will never reach the truth that tagliatelle noodles should be eight millimeters wide. To truly understand food, it must be experienced.

I think Goethe would see our food problem—our runaway appetite and our total inability to understand one of nature's most basic behaviors—as a symptom of a deeper mistake. We treat ourselves as though we are machines. It is an error we repeat, over and over.

It started in 1941, when the US government took the point of view that humans were like a line of identical but faulty toaster ovens, and all that was needed to fix them was to quietly sift some vitamins into the flour. With the barest understanding of nutrition, and not even a clue as to the true complexity of the human animal, the government believed it could correct a glaring deficiency in food with an easy and obvious fix. That's where the new road began. On its decades-long journey it has taken us to modified starches, maltodextrin, sugar alcohols, sucralose, flavorings, Simplesse, and Creamfibre 7000. We should have hit the brakes years ago. But we press on, convinced that salvation is around the next corner.

Well, here we are, around that next corner, and the new road has taken us to a place where much of what we put in our mouths hardly even qualifies as food anymore. In 2013, a software engineer who considered eating a waste of time blended the substances he deemed necessary for survival into a drink that was not only quick to consume but gave him what he believed was pinpoint control over his nutrition. The beverage, called Soylent, is an engineering marvel, featuring a cast of ingredients that have only recently come into existence: soy protein isolate, maltodextrin, high-oleic sunflower oil, artificial flavors, isomaltose, soluble corn fiber, soy lecithin, and sucralose. It is hard to imagine a more perfect example of the "we know better" approach to eating. It perfectly assumes that humans are identical machines that all run on the same fuel, that the food nature has provided is flawed and in need of correction. Soylent is the new road's ultimate destination.

Or it was. Since Soylent, the new road has taken us to a place even further removed from nature: "plant-based" meat. The makers of this industrial biochemical facsimile not only recognize their product's departure from the natural world, they embrace it. One brand is called Beyond Meat, a name that implies, with mighty hubris, that a handful of scientists are better at producing flesh than nature. The other big brand, at the present moment, is Impossible Foods—a substance that apparently defies what is possible so that humans may at last move beyond the natural world and its morbid imperfections.

When these products appeared, their apparent superiority over actual food wasn't debated so much as acclaimed. So certain were people of the deadliness of actual meat that the fake version received a spontaneous ovation. This is why we love the new road. It keeps promising salvation, and we keep believing.

If you take Goethe's position that by examining the part we can glimpse the whole, we can ask the following question: What does the food we eat today reflect back at us? When Dana Small peered deeply into sweetness, she saw not only that experiencing sweetness caused a pleasurable sensation, but that sweetness is a signal of information that suffuses our bodies and our brains. It's as though in nature, sweet foods come with their own set of operating instructions. Or consider fruit. We know that when we taste, say, a strawberry, the flavors we sense are synthesized by the plant from which the strawberry was plucked. Evolution selected a strawberry to taste like what it is: a strawberry. Its flavor is a chemical image of itself projected inside the human brain.

When we taste meat—actual, nonfake meat—what is reflected back at us? The animal, for one. A cow tastes like beef, which is distinct from lamb, which is distinct from chicken, which is distinct from pork. It is as though the brain can perceive a species' essence. We also taste the life that animal led. A deer that grazes on sagebrush tastes of sagebrush. A pig that gets fat on modern pig feed tastes different from a pig raised on pasture. This is why the Learned Brotherhood of the Tortellino stipulates there is a proper way to serve tortellini: in a broth made using a farmyard chicken. Because that chicken's life of eating bugs and seeds and leaves is reflected in a more nutritious and superior-tasting broth.

So what, then, do we see when we peer deeply into fake meat? We see a substance exquisitely engineered to taste like something that it is not. It is proudly and supremely fake. All remnants of its plant origins have been obliterated. The image it projects is designed to be illusory. This, we believe, will save us from ourselves.

For all its breathtaking scientific complexity, what the new road missed, and what it keeps missing, is Goethe's "metamorphosis" part of being alive. Human beings are not industrial widgets. Every person is in a perpetual state of ever-changing uniqueness. On the most basic level, eating is how an organism uses what is outside its body to bring the inside into balance. The new road presumed that eating was a fundamentally dumb behavior. It was sure it knew better. That was the new road's fatal mistake.

But what truly matters about Goethe is his distinctive approach to science. He didn't believe the role of the scientist was to coldly analyze data and render the world around us in numbers. He believed that it was only through experience—by seeing with the mind—that the secrets of nature could be known. He was, in that sense, the opposite of a behaviorist. Behaviorists believed the mental experience of life was private and unmeasurable. Goethe believed experience was our only true connection to the world. Pleasure wasn't a distraction, some figment of the primitive mind that clouded rational thought. It was a part of knowledge.

This unending desire to explore, to pull the blanket away from life and its mysteries, is also how Goethe approached food. Who else would travel to a foreign country in part to eat a fruit he had never tasted before? Who else would make a diary entry commending the outstanding lettuce? Who else would grow odd varieties of vegetables in his greenhouse or have his own asparagus garden?

We don't let ourselves see the world that way. We perpetually build a wall between our thinking self and our pleasure-seeking self. We cling to the faith that the cold science of nutrition can guide our eating, even though that science keeps changing and we are almost hilariously incapable of following its direction. We reduce the experience of eating to nothing more than bursts of dangerous brain chemicals.

The joy nature bestows through food is not an impediment to nutrition. It is, and should be, our guide. On some deep level, Italians never forgot what animals intuitively understand: that what tastes good is good. For too many of us, that way of eating has been lost. But I think we can learn it again.

I NEVER did figure out what makes Italians tick. I still don't know why they stuck to the old road, why they lust after the joy of eating when so many others cower in fear of it, why they never fell for the trappings of the new road but maintained their faith in the goodness of what nature provides. Italians are different now just as they were different when Goethe sat down with that family in Sicily in 1787 to make pasta. But I do know this: Italy, in its superb eccentricity, offers us a glimpse of the path we could have taken, and one that we can still take.

It's nice to imagine the old road as a footpath that wends through the Italian hills up into France, with grandmothers curing sausages in old wooden sheds and grandfathers roasting rabbits over crackling fires while sipping homemade wine. But that's not the old road. That's just a place it can take you.

The old road runs through your brain. It is a path laid down by the trillions of organisms that preceded you that lived and died by the brute circumstance of evolution. It possesses a wisdom and computational power our conscious selves are only beginning to understand. We are, alas, too stupid to understand how smart we truly are.

This behavior we call eating used to seem so simple. Now, after spending more than half my life thinking about eating and writing about eating and doing a lot of eating, I don't quite know what to make of it. Sometimes I think it is best thought of as a program, a brilliant, instantaneous functioning of some deep and ancient brain system. But then I catch myself, because programs are for machines and we are not machines. We are living beings. But I do know this: eating is propelled by a force whose roots stretch back to the days when we were slugs, and whose lines of biological code have been written, eon after eon, according to the harshest game of them all: survival.

Perhaps eating is best thought of as a performance of life itself. It is one of the best performances there is. Nature didn't create it to fool us or to kill us but to thrill us. Yet, every one of us ends up seeing a different show. I thought of those laborers in Karnataka sucking on tamarind, the Irish prisoner basking in the brutal rhapsody of six oranges, Enzo the bean farmer, that Christmas Eve dinner Anja Hilbert ate in Normandy, and the men who dress in saffron-colored robes to honor the pasta dumpling they love.

Enjoyment, rapture, "liking"—it goes by many names. It is like a god. Invisible, pure, and heavenly. It is the true object of all desires. And it sits, waiting for you, at the end of every mystery.

Acknowledgments

On September 9, 2019, a neurologist at Toronto Western Hospital named Richard Wennberg was doing his morning rounds when his attention was caught by a brain scan displayed on a wall monitor. In the middle of the image he saw a glowing V, which Wennberg recognized as "the claustrum sign." The patient was suffering from autoimmune encephalitis. His brain was being attacked by his own system.

That patient was me. If not for Dr. Wennberg's instant diagnosis, I might have suffered permanent neurological impairment, or possibly died. Without the care of the extremely talented nurses and doctors at Toronto Western, this book would not exist.

Thank you.

I wish I could thank every scientist who contributed to this book, but that is not possible. Every scientific discovery is informed by a previous discovery, which is informed by a previous discovery, and so on, stretching all the way back to when our ancestors began fashioning tools from wood and stone. I do, however, owe a special note of gratitude to a handful of researchers who spared no effort to convey the nuance and detail of their amazing research. In no particular order, they are: Kent Berridge, Ivan de Araujo, Dana Small, Kevin Hall, and Anja Hilbert.

Thank you to my editor, Julianna Haubner, whose dislike of polenta in no way impeded her superb ability to clarify my thoughts and words. It is, similarly, a privilege to work with the team of copyeditors, designers, editors, and publicists at Avid Reader Press.

I owe a special thanks to my agent, Richard Morris. Writers have a way of making every book a life and death struggle. This time, it really was one. Thank you for your loyalty and your friendship, for getting me back on my feet and seeing this thing through to the end.

Finally, thank you, Laura. Somehow you juggled three children, a cat, a puppy, and a full-time job and still found time to nurse both a husband and a manuscript to good health. I couldn't do it without you.

Bibliography

Allison, David B. "Annual Deaths Attributable to Obesity in the United States." *JAMA* 282, no. 16 (October 27, 1999): 1530. https://doi.org/10.1001/jama.282.16.1530.

Anderson, Cheryl A. M., and Lawrence J. Appel. "Dietary Modification and CVD Prevention: A Matter of Fat." *JAMA* 295, no. 6 (February 8, 2006): 693. https://doi.org/10.1001/jama.295.6.693.

Anselme, Patrick, and Mike J. F. Robinson. "What Motivates Gambling Behavior? Insight into Dopamine's Role." *Frontiers in Behavioral Neuroscience* 7 (2013). https://doi.org/10.3389/fnbeh.2013.00182.

Araujo, Ivan E. de, Albino J. Oliveira-Maia, Tatyana D. Sotnikova, Raul R. Gainetdinov, Marc G. Caron, Miguel A. L. Nicolelis, and Sidney A. Simon. "Food Reward in the Absence of Taste Receptor Signaling." *Neuron* 57, no. 6 (March 2008): 930–41. https://doi.org/10.1016/j.neuron.2008.01.032.

Astell-Burt, Thomas, Xiaoqi Feng, Karen Croteau, and Gregory S. Kolt. "Influence of Neighbourhood Ethnic Density, Diet and Physical Activity on Ethnic Differences in Weight Status: A Study of 214,807 Adults in Australia." *Social Science & Medicine* 93 (September 2013): 70–77. https://doi.org/10.1016/j.socscimed.2013.06.006.

Atkins, Robert C. *Dr. Atkins' Diet Revolution: The High Calorie Way to Stay Thin Forever*. New York: Bantam Books, 1989.

Azad, Meghan B., Ahmed M. Abou-Setta, Bhupendrasinh F. Chauhan, Rasheda Rabbani, Justin Lys, Leslie Copstein, Amrinder Mann, et al. "Nonnutritive Sweeteners and Cardiometabolic Health: A Systematic Review and Meta-Analysis of Randomized Controlled Trials and Prospective Cohort Studies." *Canadian Medical Association Journal* 189, no. 28 (July 17, 2017): E929–39. https://doi.org/10.1503/cmaj.161390.

Barnes, Richard H., Grace Fiala, Bette McGehee, and Ann Brown. "Prevention of Coprophagy in the Rat." *Journal of Nutrition* 63, no. 4 (December 1, 1957): 489–98. https://doi.org/10.1093/jn/63.4.489.

Basavaraja, H., A. Y. Hugar, S. B. Mahajanashetti, V. V. Angadi, and B. Dayakar Rao. "Kharif Sorghum in Karnataka: An Economic Analysis." *Agricultural Economic Research Review* 18, no. 2 (July–December 2005): 223–40.

Baskin, D., T. Hahn, and M. Schwartz. "Leptin Sensitive Neurons in the Hypothalamus." *Hormone and Metabolic Research* 31, no. 5 (May 1999): 345–50. https://doi.org/10.1055/s-2007-978751.

Belluz, Julia. "Why Do Dieters Succeed or Fail? The Answers Have Little to Do with Food." Vox.com, March 13, 2008.

BeMiller, James N. "One Hundred Years of Commercial Food Carbohydrates in the United States." *Journal of Agricultural and Food Chemistry* 57, no. 18 (September 23, 2009): 8125–29. https://doi.org/10.1021/jf8039236.

Berridge, Kent C. "Food Reward: Brain Substrates of Wanting and Liking." *Neuroscience and Biobehavioral Reviews* 20, no. 1 (1996): 1–25. https://doi.org/10.1016/0149-7634(95)00033-b.

———. "'Liking' and 'Wanting' Food Rewards: Brain Substrates and Roles in Eating Disorders." *Physiology & Behavior* 97, no. 5 (July 2009): 537–50. https://doi.org/10.1016/j.physbeh.2009.02.044.

Berridge, Kent C., Chao-Yi Ho, Jocelyn M. Richard, and Alexandra G. DiFeliceantonio. "The Tempted Brain Eats: Pleasure and Desire Circuits in Obesity and Eating Disorders." *Brain Research* 1350 (September 2010): 43–64. https://doi.org/10.1016/j.brainres.2010.04.003.

Berridge, Kent C., and Morten L. Kringelbach. "Pleasure Systems in the Brain." *Neuron* 86, no. 3 (May 2015): 646–64. https://doi.org/10.1016/j.neuron.2015.02.018.

Bishai, David, and Ritu Nalubola. "The History of Food Fortification in the United States: Its Relevance for Current Fortification Efforts in Developing Countries." *Economic Development and Cultural Change* 51, no. 1 (October 2002): 37–53. https://doi.org/10.1086/345361.

Blum, Sam. "Mountain Goats Are Being Airlifted out of a National Park Because They Crave Human Pee." *Popular Mechanics*, September 29, 2018.

Boakes, R. A. "Performance on Learning to Associate a Stimulus with Positive Reinforcement." In *Operant-Pavlovian Interactions*, edited by Hank Davis and Harry M. B. Hurwitz. Hillsdale, NJ: L. Erlbaum Associates, 1977.

Bollet, A. J. "Politics and Pellagra: The Epidemic of Pellagra in the U.S. in the Early Twentieth Century." *Yale Journal of Biology and Medicine* 65, no. 3 (June 1992): 211–21.

Booth, Helen P., Judith Charlton, and Martin C. Gulliford. "Socioeconomic Inequality in Morbid Obesity with Body Mass Index More than 40 Kg/M2 in the United States and England." *SSM—Population Health* 3 (December 2017): 172–78. https://doi.org/10.1016/j.ssmph.2016.12.012.

Boots, Samantha B., Marika Tiggemann, and Nadia Corsini. "Eating in the Absence of Hunger in Young Children: The Role of Maternal Feeding Strategies." *Appetite* 130 (November 2018): 45–49. https://doi.org/10.1016/j.appet.2018.07.024.

Bortoft, Henri, and Johann Wolfgang von Goethe. *The Wholeness of Nature: Goethe's Way of Science*. Edinburgh: Floris Books (u.a.), 1996.

Bratke, Heiko, Ingvild Særvold Bruserud, Bente Brannsether, Jörg Aßmus, Robert Bjerknes, Mathieu Roelants, and Pétur B. Júlíusson. "Timing of Menarche in Norwegian Girls: Associations with Body Mass Index, Waist Circumference and Skinfold Thickness." *BMC Pediatrics* 17, no. 1 (December 2017): 138. https://doi.org/10.1186/s12887-017-0893-x.

Bray, George A. "Luxuskonsumption—Myth or Reality?" *Obesity Research* 3, no. 5 (September 1995): 491–95. https://doi.org/10.1002/j.1550-8528.1995.tb00180.x.

Brown, Paul L., and Herbert M. Jenkins. "Auto-Shaping of the Pigeon's Key-Peck." *Journal of the Experimental Analysis of Behavior* 11, no. 1 (January 1968): 1–8. https://doi.org/10.1901/jeab.1968.11-1.

Buga, Alex, Madison L. Kackley, Christopher D. Crabtree, Teryn N. Sapper, Lauren Mccabe, Brandon Fell, Rich A. LaFountain, et al. "The Effects of a 6-Week Controlled, Hypocaloric Ketogenic Diet, With and Without Exogenous Ketone Salts, on Body Composition Responses." *Frontiers in Nutrition* 8 (March 24, 2021): 618520. https://doi.org/10.3389/fnut.2021.618520.

Caballero, Benjamin, Paul M. Finglas, and Fidel Toldrá, eds. *Encyclopedia of Food and Health*. Amsterdam and Boston: Academic Press, an imprint of Elsevier, 2016.

Cabanac, M., R. Duclaux, and N. H. Spector. "Sensory Feedback in Regulation of Body Weight: Is There a Ponderostat?" *Nature* 229, no. 5280 (January 1971): 125–27. https://doi.org/10.1038/229125a0.

Cabanac, Michel. *The Fifth Influence: The Dialectics of Pleasure*. Bloomington, IN: iUniverse, 2010.

———. *The Quest for Pleasure*. Montreal: Liber, 1999.

Cantor, Jonathan, Alejandro Torres, Courtney Abrams, and Brian Elbel. "Five Years Later: Awareness of New York City's Calorie Labels Declined, with No Changes in Calories Purchased." *Health Affairs* 34, no. 11 (November 2015): 1893–900. https://doi.org/10.1377/hlthaff.2015.0623.

Cantu-Jungles, Thaisa, Lacey McCormack, James Slaven, Maribeth Slebodnik, and Heather Eicher-Miller. "A Meta-Analysis to Determine the Impact of Restaurant Menu Labeling on Calories and Nutrients (Ordered or Consumed) in U.S. Adults." *Nutrients* 9, no. 10 (September 30, 2017): 1088. https://doi.org/10.3390/nu9101088.

Carpenter, Kenneth J. *The History of Scurvy and Vitamin C*. Cambridge, UK: Cambridge University Press, 2003.

Castro, Daniel C., Shannon L. Cole, and Kent C. Berridge. "Lateral Hypothalamus, Nucleus Accumbens, and Ventral Pallidum Roles in Eating and Hunger: Interactions between Homeostatic and Reward Circuitry." *Frontiers in Systems Neuroscience* 9 (2015): 90. https://doi.org/10.3389/fnsys.2015.00090.

Chandrashekar, Janakiram, K. R. Thankappan, and K. R. Sundaram. "Severe Dental Fluorosis among Jowar Consumers in India." *Community Dentistry and Oral Epidemiology* 38, no. 6 (December 2010): 559–67. https://doi.org/10.1111/j.1600-0528.2010.00564.x.

Childress, Anna Rose, Ronald N. Ehrman, Ze Wang, Yin Li, Nathan Sciortino, Jonathan Hakun, William Jens, et al. "Prelude to Passion: Limbic Activation by 'Unseen' Drug and Sexual Cues." Edited by Aldo Rustichini. *PLoS ONE* 3, no. 1 (January 30, 2008): e1506. https://doi.org/10.1371/journal.pone.0001506.

Choubisa, S. L. "Natural Amelioration of Fluoride Toxicity (Fluorosis) in Goats and Sheep." *Current Science* 99 (2010): 1331–32.

Choubisa, S. L., G. V. Mishra, Zulfiya Sheikh, B. Bhardwaj, P. Mali, and V. J. Jaroli. "Food, Fluoride, and Fluorosis in Domestic Ruminants in the Dungarpur District of Rajasthan, India." *Fluoride* 44, no. 2 (April–June 2011): 70–76.

Chow, Carson C., and Kevin D. Hall. "Short- and Long-Term Energy Intake Patterns and Their Implications for Human Body Weight Regulation." *Physiology & Behavior* 134 (July 2014): 60–65. https://doi.org/10.1016/j.physbeh.2014.02.044.

Corriher, Shirley O. "Science of Starch for the Perfect Sauce." *South Forida Sun-Sentinel*, May 18, 2006.

Coy, Peter. "Discovery of Simplessse Was an Accident." Associated Press, January 28, 1988.

Dalenberg, Jelle R., Barkha P. Patel, Raphael Denis, Maria G. Veldhuizen, Yuko Nakamura, Petra C. Vinke, Serge Luquet, and Dana M. Small. "Short-Term Consumption of Sucralose with, but Not without, Carbohydrate Impairs Neural and Metabolic Sensitivity to Sugar in Humans." *Cell*

Metabolism 31, no. 3 (March 2020): 493–502.e7. https://doi.org/10.1016 /j.cmet.2020.01.014.

Danubio, Maria Enrica, Elisa Amicone, and Rita Vargiu. "Height and BMI of Italian Immigrants to the USA, 1908–1970." *Economics & Human Biology* 3, no. 1 (March 2005): 33–43. https://doi.org/10.1016/j.ehb.2004.11.001.

Davis, Caroline A., Robert D. Levitan, Caroline Reid, Jacqueline C. Carter, Allan S. Kaplan, Karen A. Patte, Nicole King, Claire Curtis, and James L. Kennedy. "Dopamine for 'Wanting' and Opioids for 'Liking': A Comparison of Obese Adults with and without Binge Eating." *Obesity* 17, no. 6 (June 2009): 1220–25. https://doi.org/10.1038/oby.2009.52.

Deaderick, William, and Loyd Thompson. "The Endemic Diseases of the Southern States." *Journal of the American Medical Association* 57, no. 7 (August 12, 1916): 537. https://doi.org/10.1001/jama.1916.02590070061029.

DeKleine, William. "Recent Trends in Pellagra." *American Journal of Public Health* 27, no. 6 (June 1937): 595–99.

Demos, K. E., T. F. Heatherton, and W. M. Kelley. "Individual Differences in Nucleus Accumbens Activity to Food and Sexual Images Predict Weight Gain and Sexual Behavior." *Journal of Neuroscience* 32, no. 16 (April 18, 2012): 5549–52. https://doi.org/10.1523/JNEUROSCI.5958-11.2012.

Dietz, W. H. "Does Hunger Cause Obesity?" *Pediatrics* 95, no. 5 (May 1995): 766–67.

Dietz, W. H., and S. L. Gortmaker. "Do We Fatten Our Children at the Television Set? Obesity and Television Viewing in Children and Adolescents." *Pediatrics* 75, no. 5 (May 1985): 807–12.

Drewnowski, A., J. Buszkiewicz, A. Aggarwal, A. Cook, and A. V. Moudon. "A New Method to Visualize Obesity Prevalence in Seattle-King County at the Census Block Level: Mapping Obesity at the Census Block." *Obesity Science & Practice* 4, no. 1 (February 2018): 14–19. https://doi .org/10.1002/osp4.144.

Dror, Otniel E. "Cold War 'Super-Pleasure': Insatiability, Self-Stimulation, and the Postwar Brain." *Osiris* 31, no. 1 (July 2016): 227–49. https://doi .org/10.1086/688162.

Dyer, I. A., J. L. Krider, and W. E. Carroll. "Known and Unidentified Factors Supplement a Corn-Soybean Meal Ration for Weanling Pigs in Drylot." *Journal of Animal Science* 8, no. 4 (November 1, 1949): 541–49. https:// doi.org/10.2527/jas1949.84541x.

Edholm, O. G., J. M. Adam, M. J. R. Healy, H. S. Wolff, R. Goldsmith, and T. W. Best. "Food Intake and Energy Expenditure of Army Recruits." *British Journal of Nutrition* 24, no. 4 (December 1970): 1091–107. https://doi .org/10.1079/BJN19700112.

"Effectiveness of Food Fortification in the United States: The Case of Pellagra." *American Journal of Public Health* 90, no. 5 (May 2000): 727–38. https://doi.org/10.2105/AJPH.90.5.727.

El-Siddig, K. *Tamarind: Tamarindus indica L.* Southampton, UK: International Centre for Underutilised Crops, University of Southampton, 2006.

Elvehjem, C. A., R. J. Madden, F. M. Strong, and D. W. Woolley. "Relation of Nicotinic Acid and Nicotinic Acid Amide to Canine Black Tongue." *Journal of the American Chemical Society* 59, no. 9 (September 1937): 1767–68. https://doi.org/10.1021/ja01288a509.

Epstein, Leonard H., Noelle Jankowiak, Kelly D. Fletcher, Katelyn A. Carr, Chantal Nederkoorn, Hollie A. Raynor, and Eric Finkelstein. "Women Who Are Motivated to Eat and Discount the Future Are More Obese: BMI and Reinforcement Pathology." *Obesity* 22, no. 6 (June 2014): 1394–99. https://doi.org/10.1002/oby.20661.

Evans, Andrew H., Regina Katzenschlager, Dominic Paviour, John D. O'Sullivan, Silke Appel, Andrew D. Lawrence, and Andrew J. Lees. "Punding in Parkinson's Disease: Its Relation to the Dopamine Dysregulation Syndrome." *Movement Disorders* 19, no. 4 (April 2004): 397–405. https://doi.org/10.1002/mds.20045.

Ferreira, Jozélia G., Luis A. Tellez, Xueying Ren, Catherine W. Yeckel, and Ivan E. de Araujo. "Regulation of Fat Intake in the Absence of Flavour Signalling: Fat Intake in the Absence of Flavour." *Journal of Physiology* 590, no. 4 (February 15, 2012): 953–72. https://doi.org/10.1113/jphysiol.2011.218289.

Fidanza, Flaminio, Adalberta Alberti, and Daniela Fruttini. "The Nicotera Diet: The Reference Italian Mediterranean Diet." In *World Review of Nutrition and Dietetics*, edited by A. P. Simopoulos, 115–21. Basel: Karger, 2005. https://doi.org/10.1159/000088278.

Finucane, Mariel M., Gretchen A. Stevens, Melanie J. Cowan, Goodarz Danaei, John K. Lin, Christopher J. Paciorek, Gitanjali M. Singh, et al. "National, Regional, and Global Trends in Body-Mass Index since 1980: Systematic Analysis of Health Examination Surveys and Epidemiological Studies with 960 Country-Years and 9·1 Million Participants." *Lancet* 377, no. 9765 (February 2011): 557–67. https://doi.org/10.1016/S0140-6736(10)62037-5.

Fiorillo, Christopher D., Philippe N. Tobler, and Wolfram Schultz. "Discrete Coding of Reward Probability and Uncertainty by Dopamine Neurons." *Science* (New York, NY) 299, no. 5614 (March 21, 2003): 1898–1902. https://doi.org/10.1126/science.1077349.

Fisher, Jennifer Orlet, and Leann Lipps Birch. "Restricting Access to Palatable Foods Affects Children's Behavioral Response, Food Selection, and Intake." *American Journal of Clinical Nutrition* 69, no. 6 (June 1, 1999): 1264–72. https://doi.org/10.1093/ajcn/69.6.1264.

Fleissner, Jennifer L. "Earth-Eating, Addiction, Nostalgia: Charles Chesnutt's Diasporic Regionalism." *Studies in Romanticism* 49, no. 2 (2010): 313–36.

Forkman, B. A. "The Effect of Uncertainty on the Food Intake of the Mongolian Gerbil." *Behaviour* 124, no. 3–4 (1993): 197–206. https://doi.org/10.1163/156853993X00579.

Fothergill, Erin, Juen Guo, Lilian Howard, Jennifer C. Kerns, Nicolas D. Knuth, Robert Brychta, Kong Y. Chen, et al. "Persistent Metabolic Adaptation 6 Years after 'The Biggest Loser' Competition: Persistent Metabolic Adaptation." *Obesity* 24, no. 8 (August 2016): 1612–19. https://doi.org/10.1002/oby.21538.

Frank, Lawrence D., Martin A. Andresen, and Thomas L. Schmid. "Obesity Relationships with Community Design, Physical Activity, and Time Spent in Cars." *American Journal of Preventive Medicine* 27, no. 2 (August 2004): 87–96. https://doi.org/10.1016/j.amepre.2004.04.011.

Furedi, Frank. "The Media's First Moral Panic." *History Today* 65, no. 11 (2015).

Gallus, S., P. Colombo, V. Scarpino, P. Zuccaro, E. Negri, G. Apolone, and C. La Vecchia. "Overweight and Obesity in Italian Adults 2004, and an Overview of Trends since 1983." *European Journal of Clinical Nutrition* 60, no. 10 (October 2006): 1174–79. https://doi.org/10.1038/sj.ejcn.1602433.

Gallus, Silvano, Alessandra Lugo, Bojana Murisic, Cristina Bosetti, Paolo Boffetta, and Carlo La Vecchia. "Overweight and Obesity in 16 European Countries." *European Journal of Nutrition* 54, no. 5 (August 2015): 679–89. https://doi.org/10.1007/s00394-014-0746-4.

Gallus, Silvano, Anna Odone, Alessandra Lugo, Cristina Bosetti, Paolo Colombo, Piergiorgio Zuccaro, and Carlo La Vecchia. "Overweight and Obesity Prevalence and Determinants in Italy: An Update to 2010." *European Journal of Nutrition* 52, no. 2 (March 2013): 677–85. https://doi.org/10.1007/s00394-012-0372-y.

Gardner, Christopher D., John F. Trepanowski, Liana C. Del Gobbo, Michelle E. Hauser, Joseph Rigdon, John P. A. Ioannidis, Manisha Desai, and Abby C. King. "Effect of Low-Fat vs Low-Carbohydrate Diet on 12-Month Weight Loss in Overweight Adults and the Association with Genotype Pattern or Insulin Secretion: The DIETFITS Randomized Clinical Trial." *JAMA* 319, no. 7 (February 20, 2018): 667–79. https://doi.org/10.1001/jama.2018.0245.

Garine, I., and G. Koppert. "Guru-Fattening Sessions among the Massa." *Ecology of Modern Food and Nutrition* 25 (1991): 1–28.

Gebauer, Line, Morten L. Kringelbach, and Peter Vuust. "Ever-Changing Cycles of Musical Pleasure: The Role of Dopamine and Anticipation." *Psychomusicology: Music, Mind, and Brain* 22, no. 2 (December 2012): 152–67. https://doi.org/10.1037/a0031126.

Ginnaio, Monica. "La pellagre en Italie à la fin du XIXe siècle: Les effets d'une maladie de carence." *Population* 66, no. 3–4 (2011): 671–98. https://doi.org/10.3917/popu.1103.0671.

Goethe, Johann Wolfgang von, W. H. Auden, and Elizabeth Mayer. *Italian Journey (1786–1788)*. Penguin Classics 16. London: Penguin, 1970.

Goethe, Johann Wolfgang von, and Karl Richter. *Sämtliche Werke Nach Epochen Seines Schaffens, Münchner Ausgabe*. München: C. Hanser, 1985.

Goldberger, Joseph. "Public Health Reports: The Transmissibility of Pellagra." *Nutrition Reviews* 31, no. 6 (April 27, 2009): 184–86. https://doi.org/10.1111/j.1753-4887.1973.tb05173.x.

Goldberger, Joseph, C. H. Wariu, and David G. Willets. "The Prevention of Pellagra: A Test of Diet among Institutional Inmates." *Nutrition Reviews* 31, no. 5 (April 27, 2009): 152–53. https://doi.org/10.1111/j.1753-4887.1973.tb05159.x.

"Goldberger: An Unremitting Struggle to Conquer Pellagra." *Hospital Practice* 13, no. 3 (March 1978): 136, 141–42, 147–48 passim. https://doi.org/10.1080/21548331.1978.11707302.

Green, Erin, and Claire Murphy. "Altered Processing of Sweet Taste in the Brain of Diet Soda Drinkers." *Physiology & Behavior* 107, no. 4 (November 2012): 560–67. https://doi.org/10.1016/j.physbeh.2012.05.006.

Haddix, Carol. "That Phenomenon Simplesse Supplies the Feeling of Fat." *Chicago Tribune*, February 4, 1988.

Hall, K. D. "A Review of the Carbohydrate-Insulin Model of Obesity." *European Journal of Clinical Nutrition* 71, no. 3 (March 2017): 323–26. https://doi.org/10.1038/ejcn.2016.260.

Hall, Kevin D., Thomas Bemis, Robert Brychta, Kong Y. Chen, Amber Courville, Emma J. Crayner, Stephanie Goodwin, et al. "Calorie for Calorie, Dietary Fat Restriction Results in More Body Fat Loss than Carbohydrate Restriction in People with Obesity." *Cell Metabolism* 22, no. 3 (September 2015): 427–36. https://doi.org/10.1016/j.cmet.2015.07.021.

Hall, Kevin D., Kong Y. Chen, Juen Guo, Yan Y. Lam, Rudolph L. Leibel, Laurel E. S. Mayer, Marc L. Reitman, et al. "Energy Expenditure and Body Composition Changes after an Isocaloric Ketogenic Diet in Overweight and Obese Men." *American Journal of Clinical Nutrition* 104, no. 2 (August 2016): 324–33. https://doi.org/10.3945/ajcn.116.133561.

Hall, Kevin D., and Juen Guo. "Obesity Energetics: Body Weight Regulation and the Effects of Diet Composition." *Gastroenterology* 152, no. 7 (May 2017): 1718–27.e3. https://doi.org/10.1053/j.gastro.2017.01.052.

Heath, Robert G. "Electrical Self-Stimulation of the Brain in Man." *American Journal of Psychiatry* 120, no. 6 (December 1963): 571–77. https://doi .org/10.1176/ajp.120.6.571.

Hilbert, Anja, Marie Blume, David Petroff, Petra Neuhaus, Evelyn Smith, Phillipa J Hay, and Claudia Hübner. "Group Cognitive Remediation Therapy for Adults with Obesity Prior to Behavioural Weight Loss Treatment: Study Protocol for a Randomised Controlled Superiority Study (CRT Study)." *BMJ Open* 8, no. 9 (September 2018): e022616. https://doi .org/10.1136/bmjopen-2018-022616.

Howard, Barbara V., Linda Van Horn, Judith Hsia, JoAnn E. Manson, Marcia L. Stefanick, Sylvia Wassertheil-Smoller, Lewis H. Kuller, et al. "Low-Fat Dietary Pattern and Risk of Cardiovascular Disease: The Women's Health Initiative Randomized Controlled Dietary Modification Trial." *JAMA* 295, no. 6 (February 8, 2006): 655. https://doi.org/10.1001/jama .295.6.655.

Hu, Sumei, Lu Wang, Jacques Togo, Dengbao Yang, Yanchao Xu, Yingga Wu, Alex Douglas, and John R. Speakman. "The Carbohydrate-Insulin Model Does Not Explain the Impact of Varying Dietary Macronutrients on the Body Weight and Adiposity of Mice." *Molecular Metabolism* 32 (February 2020): 27–43. https://doi.org/10.1016/j.molmet.2019.11.010.

"Human Gastric Function: An Experimental Study of a Man and His Stomach." *Journal of the American Medical Association* 135, no. 3 (September 20, 1947): 195. https://doi.org/10.1001/jama.1947.02890030063030.

Hundley, J. M. "Influence of Fructose and Other Carbohydrates on the Niacin Requirement of the Rat." *Journal of Biological Chemistry* 181, no. 1 (November 1949): 1–9.

Hutchinson, H. D., S. W. Terrill, A. H. Jensen, D. E. Becker, and H. W. Norton. "Comparison of Free-Choice and Complete Rations for Growing-Finishing Pigs on Pasture and Drylot." *Journal of Animal Science* 16, no. 3 (1957): 562–67. https://doi.org/10.2527/1957.163562x.

Institute of Medicine (US), eds. *Dietary Reference Intakes for Thiamin, Riboflavin, Niacin, Vitamin B$_6$, Folate, Vitamin B$_{12}$, Pantothenic Acid, Biotin, and Choline.* Washington, DC: National Academy Press, 1998.

Jansson, John-Olov, Vilborg Palsdottir, Daniel A. Hägg, Erik Schéle, Suzanne

L. Dickson, Fredrik Anesten, Tina Bake, et al. "Body Weight Homeostat That Regulates Fat Mass Independently of Leptin in Rats and Mice." *Proceedings of the National Academy of Sciences* 115, no. 2 (January 9, 2018): 427–32. https://doi.org/10.1073/pnas.1715687114.

Jiang, P., J. Josue, X. Li, D. Glaser, W. Li, J. G. Brand, R. F. Margolskee, D. R. Reed, and G. K. Beauchamp. "Major Taste Loss in Carnivorous Mammals." *Proceedings of the National Academy of Sciences* 109, no. 13 (March 27, 2012): 4956–61. https://doi.org/10.1073/pnas.1118360109.

Kahneman, Daniel. *Thinking, Fast and Slow*. New York: Farrar, Straus and Giroux, 2013.

Kahneman, Daniel, and Amos Tversky. "Prospect Theory: An Analysis of Decision under Risk." *Econometrica* 47, no. 2 (March 1979): 263. https://doi.org/10.2307/1914185.

Kalm, Leah M., and Richard D. Semba. "They Starved So That Others Be Better Fed: Remembering Ancel Keys and the Minnesota Experiment." *Journal of Nutrition* 135, no. 6 (June 1, 2005): 1347–52. https://doi.org/10.1093/jn/135.6.1347.

Kerns, Jennifer C., Juen Guo, Erin Fothergill, Lilian Howard, Nicolas D. Knuth, Robert Brychta, Kong Y. Chen, Monica C. Skarulis, Peter J. Walter, and Kevin D. Hall. "Increased Physical Activity Associated with Less Weight Regain Six Years after 'The Biggest Loser' Competition." *Obesity* (Silver Spring, MD) 25, no. 11 (November 2017): 1838–43. https://doi.org/10.1002/oby.21986.

Khandare, A. L., G. S. Rao, and N. Lakshmaiah. "Effect of Tamarind Ingestion on Fluoride Excretion in Humans." *European Journal of Clinical Nutrition* 56, no. 1 (January 2002): 82–85. https://doi.org/10.1038/sj.ejcn.1601287.

Khandare, Arjun, P. Uday Kumar, and Nakka Lakshmaiah. "Beneficial Effect of Tamarind Ingestion on Fluoride Toxicity in Dogs." *Fluoride* 33, no. 1 (November 1999): 33–38.

Khandare, Arjun L., P. Uday Kumar , Rao G. Shanker, K. Venkaiah, and N. Lakshmaiah. "Additional Beneficial Effect of Tamarind Ingestion over Defluoridated Water Supply to Adolescent Boys in a Fluorotic Area." *Nutrition* 20, no. 5 (May 2004): 433–36. https://doi.org/10.1016/j.nut.2004.01.007.

Khandare, Arjun, Komal Rasaputra, Indrapal Meshram, and Rao Shankar. "Effects of Smoking, Use of Aluminium Utensils, and Tamarind Consumption on Fluorosis in a Fluorotic Village of Andhra Pradesh, India." *Fluoride* 43, no. 2 (2010): 128–33.

Kilmister, C. W. *The Environment in Modern Physics: A Study in Relativistic Mechanics*. New York: American Elsevier, 1965.

Kim, W. W., J. L. Kelsay, J. T. Judd, M. W. Marshall, W. Mertz, and E. S. Prather. "Evaluation of Long-Term Dietary Intakes of Adults Consuming Self-Selected Diets." *American Journal of Clinical Nutrition* 40, no. 6 (December 1, 1984): 1327–32. https://doi.org/10.1093/ajcn/40.6.1327.

Kimenju, Simon C, Ramona Rischke, Stephan Klasen, and Matin Qaim. "Do Supermarkets Contribute to the Obesity Pandemic in Developing Countries?" *Public Health Nutrition* 18, no. 17 (December 2015): 3224–33. https://doi.org/10.1017/S1368980015000919.

Kolata, Gina Bari. *Rethinking Thin: The New Science of Weight Loss—and the Myths and Realities of Dieting.* New York: Picador/Farrar, Straus and Giroux, 2008.

Kraut, Alan. "Dr. Joseph Goldberger & the War on Pellagra." Office of NIH History & Stetten Museum, National Institutes of Health, n.d. https://history.nih.gov/pages/viewpage.action?pageId=8883184.

Kruif, Paul de. *The Fight for Life.* New York: Brace, 1937.

Kuijt, I., and B. Finlayson. "Evidence for Food Storage and Predomestication Granaries 11,000 Years Ago in the Jordan Valley." *Proceedings of the National Academy of Sciences* 106, no. 27 (July 7, 2009): 10966–70. https://doi.org/10.1073/pnas.0812764106.

Lauria, Laura, Angela Spinelli, Marta Buoncristiano, and Paola Nardone. "Decline of Childhood Overweight and Obesity in Italy from 2008 to 2016: Results from 5 Rounds of the Population-Based Surveillance System." *BMC Public Health* 19, no. 1 (December 2019): 618. https://doi.org/10.1186/s12889-019-6946-3.

Lee, Edwin. *Observations on the Principal Medical Institutions & Practice of France, Italy, & Germany: With Notices of the Universities and Cases from Hospital Practice.* Philadelphia: Haswell, Barrington and Haswell, 1837.

Lee, Yujin, Dariush Mozaffarian, Stephen Sy, Junxiu Liu, Parke E. Wilde, Matti Marklund, Shafika Abrahams-Gessel, Thomas A. Gaziano, and Renata Micha. "Health Impact and Cost-Effectiveness of Volume, Tiered, and Absolute Sugar Content Sugar-Sweetened Beverage Tax Policies in the United States: A Microsimulation Study." *Circulation* 142, no. 6 (August 11, 2020): 523–34. https://doi.org/10.1161/CIRCULATIONAHA.119.042956.

Leibel, R. L., M. Rosenbaum, and J. Hirsch. "Changes in Energy Expenditure Resulting from Altered Body Weight." *The New England Journal of Medicine* 332, no. 10 (March 9, 1995): 621–28. https://doi.org/10.1056/NEJM199503093321001.

Lewis, Michael. *The Undoing Project: A Friendship That Changed Our Minds.* New York: W. W. Norton, 2016.

Lim, Elizabeth X., Ciarán G. Forde, and Bobby K. Cheon. "Low Subjective Socioeconomic Status Alters Taste-Based Perceptual Sensitivity to the Energy Density of Beverages." *Physiology & Behavior* 223 (September 2020): 112989. https://doi.org/10.1016/j.physbeh.2020.112989.

Lioret, S., B. Maire, J.-L. Volatier, and M.-A. Charles. "Child Overweight in France and Its Relationship with Physical Activity, Sedentary Behaviour and Socioeconomic Status." *European Journal of Clinical Nutrition* 61, no. 4 (April 2007): 509–16. https://doi.org/10.1038/sj.ejcn.1602538.

Ludwig, David S., and Cara B. Ebbeling. "The Carbohydrate-Insulin Model of Obesity: Beyond 'Calories In, Calories Out.'" *JAMA Internal Medicine* 178, no. 8 (August 1, 2018): 1098. https://doi.org/10.1001/jamainternmed.2018.2933.

Malvaez, Melissa, Christine Shieh, Michael D. Murphy, Venuz Y. Greenfield, and Kate M. Wassum. "Distinct Cortical-Amygdala Projections Drive Reward Value Encoding and Retrieval." *Nature Neuroscience* 22, no. 5 (May 2019): 762–69. https://doi.org/10.1038/s41593-019-0374-7.

Mann, Traci, A. Janet Tomiyama, Erika Westling, Ann-Marie Lew, Barbra Samuels, and Jason Chatman. "Medicare's Search for Effective Obesity Treatments: Diets Are Not the Answer." *American Psychologist* 62, no. 3 (2007): 220–33. https://doi.org/10.1037/0003-066X.62.3.220.

Marks, H. M. "Epidemiologists Explain Pellagra: Gender, Race, and Political Economy in the Work of Edgar Sydenstricker." *Journal of the History of Medicine and Allied Sciences* 58, no. 1 (January 1, 2003): 34–55. https://doi.org/10.1093/jhmas/58.1.34.

Marques-Vidal, Pedro, Peter Vollenweider, Gérard Waeber, and Fred Paccaud. "Prevalence of Overweight and Obesity among Migrants in Switzerland: Association with Country of Origin." *Public Health Nutrition* 14, no. 7 (July 2011): 1148–56. https://doi.org/10.1017/S1368980011000103.

Maruthamuthu, M., and Venkatanarayana Reddy. "Binding of Fluoride with Tamarind Gel." *Fluoride* 20, no. 3 (July 1987): 109.

Mason, David. "On *Atrophia a Ventriculo* (*Mal d'Estomac*) or Dirt-Eating." *Edinburgh Medical and Surgical Journal* 39, no. 115 (April 1, 1833): 289–96.

McDowell, Lee. *Vitamin History, the Early Years*. Sarasota, FL: First Edition Design, 2013.

McMillen, W. N., R. W. Luecke, and F. Thorp. "The Effect of Liberal B-Vitamin Supplementation on Growth of Weanling Pigs Fed Rations Containing a Variety of Feedstuffs." *Journal of Animal Science* 8, no. 4 (November 1, 1949): 518–23. https://doi.org/10.2527/jas1949.84518x.

Meyers, Andrew W., Albert J. Stunkard, Milton Coll, and Christine J. Cooke. "Stairs, Escalators, and Obesity." *Behavior Modification* 4, no. 3 (July 1980): 355–59. https://doi.org/10.1177/014544558043005.

Miao, Diana, Sera L. Young, and Christopher D. Golden. "A Meta-Analysis of Pica and Micronutrient Status: Pica and Micronutrient Meta-Analysis." *American Journal of Human Biology* 27, no. 1 (January 2015): 84–93. https://doi.org/10.1002/ajhb.22598.

Mitchel, John. *Jail Journal . . . : With an Introductory Narrative of Transactions in Ireland.* Dublin: University Press of Ireland, 1982.

Moan, Charles E., and Robert G. Heath. "Septal Stimulation for the Initiation of Heterosexual Behavior in a Homosexual Male." *Journal of Behavior Therapy and Experimental Psychiatry* 3, no. 1 (March 1972): 23–30. https://doi.org/10.1016/0005-7916(72)90029-8.

Morabia, Alfredo. "Joseph Goldberger's Research on the Prevention of Pellagra." *Journal of the Royal Society of Medicine* 101, no. 11 (November 1, 2008): 566–68. https://doi.org/10.1258/jrsm.2008.08k010.

Morland, Kimberly, Ana V. Diez Roux, and Steve Wing. "Supermarkets, Other Food Stores, and Obesity." *American Journal of Preventive Medicine* 30, no. 4 (April 2006): 333–39. https://doi.org/10.1016/j.amepre.2005.11.003.

Moskowitz, H., V. Kumaraiah, K. Sharma, H. Jacobs, and S. Sharma. "Cross-Cultural Differences in Simple Taste Preferences." *Science* 190, no. 4220 (December 19, 1975): 1217–18. https://doi.org/10.1126/science.1198109.

National Research Council (US), ed. *Nutrient Requirements of Swine.* 11th rev. ed. Washington, DC: National Academies Press, 2012.

Nettle, Daniel, Clare Andrews, and Melissa Bateson. "Food Insecurity as a Driver of Obesity in Humans: The Insurance Hypothesis." *Behavioral and Brain Sciences* 40 (2017): e105. https://doi.org/10.1017/S0140525X16000947.

O'Dea, Jennifer A., and Michael J. Dibley. "Obesity Increase among Low SES Australian Schoolchildren between 2000 and 2006: Time for Preventive Interventions to Target Children from Low Income Schools?" *International Journal of Public Health* 55, no. 3 (June 2010): 185–92. https://doi.org/10.1007/s00038-009-0079-x.

Olds, James. "Pleasure Centers in the Brain." *Scientific American* 195, no. 4 (1956): 105–17.

Otto, John Solomon. *The Final Frontiers, 1880–1930: Settling the Southern Bottomlands.* Contributions in American History, no. 183. Westport, CT: Greenwood Press, 1999.

Pannia, Emanuela, Clara E. Cho, Ruslan Kubant, Diana Sánchez-Hernández, Pedro S. P. Huot, Diptendu Chatterjee, Alison Fleming, and G. Harvey

Anderson. "A High Multivitamin Diet Fed to Wistar Rat Dams during Pregnancy Increases Maternal Weight Gain Later in Life and Alters Homeostatic, Hedonic and Peripheral Regulatory Systems of Energy Balance." *Behavioural Brain Research* 278 (February 2015): 1–11. https://doi.org/10.1016/j.bbr.2014.09.019.

Park, Yong-Moon Mark, Alexandra J. White, Chandra L. Jackson, Clarice R. Weinberg, and Dale P. Sandler. "Association of Exposure to Artificial Light at Night While Sleeping with Risk of Obesity in Women." *JAMA Internal Medicine* 179, no. 8 (August 1, 2019): 1061. https://doi.org/10.1001/jamainternmed.2019.0571.

Pasquet, P., and M. Apfelbaum. "Recovery of Initial Body Weight and Composition after Long-Term Massive Overfeeding in Men." *American Journal of Clinical Nutrition* 60, no. 6 (December 1994): 861–63. https://doi.org/10.1093/ajcn/60.6.861.

Peck, Trevor Richard. *Light from Ancient Campfires: Archaeological Evidence for Native Lifeways on the Northern Plains*. Edmonton, Canada: AU Press, 2011.

Polidori, David, Arjun Sanghvi, Randy J. Seeley, and Kevin D. Hall. "How Strongly Does Appetite Counter Weight Loss? Quantification of the Feedback Control of Human Energy Intake: Feedback Control of Human Energy Intake." *Obesity* 24, no. 11 (November 2016): 2289–95. https://doi.org/10.1002/oby.21653.

Politis, Marios, Clare Loane, Kit Wu, Sean S. O'Sullivan, Zoe Woodhead, Lorenzo Kiferle, Andrew D. Lawrence, Andrew J. Lees, and Paola Piccini. "Neural Response to Visual Sexual Cues in Dopamine Treatment-Linked Hypersexuality in Parkinson's Disease." *Brain* 136, no. 2 (February 2013): 400–411. https://doi.org/10.1093/brain/aws326.

Rachmilewitz, M., and H. I. Glueck. "Treatment of Pellagra with Nicotinic Acid." *BMJ* 2, no. 4049 (August 13, 1938): 346–48. https://doi.org/10.1136/bmj.2.4049.346.

Rajakumar, K. "Pellagra in the United States: A Historical Perspective." *Southern Medical Journal* 93, no. 3 (March 2000): 272–77.

Real, D. E., J. L. Nelssen, J. A. Unruh, M. D. Tokach, R. D. Goodband, S. S. Dritz, J. M. DeRouchey, and E. Alonso. "Effects of Increasing Dietary Niacin on Growth Performance and Meat Quality in Finishing Pigs Reared in Two Different Environments." *Journal of Animal Science* 80, no. 12 (December 1, 2002): 3203–10. https://doi.org/10.2527/2002.80123203x.

Ren, Xueying, Jozélia G. Ferreira, Ligang Zhou, Sara J. Shammah-Lagnado, Catherine W. Yeckel, and Ivan E. de Araujo. "Nutrient Selection in the

Absence of Taste Receptor Signaling." *Journal of Neuroscience: The Official Journal of the Society for Neuroscience* 30, no. 23 (June 9, 2010): 8012–23. https://doi.org/10.1523/JNEUROSCI.5749-09.2010.

Reza-López, Sandra A., G. Harvey Anderson, Ignatius M. Y. Szeto, Ameer Y. Taha, and David W. L. Ma. "High Vitamin Intake by Wistar Rats during Pregnancy Alters Tissue Fatty Acid Concentration in the Offspring Fed an Obesogenic Diet." *Metabolism* 58, no. 5 (May 2009): 722–30. https://doi.org/10.1016/j.metabol.2009.01.014.

Richter, Curt P., and Clarence D. Hawkes. "The Dependence of the Carbohydrate, Fat and Protein Appetite of Rats on the Various Components of the Vitamin B Complex." *American Journal of Physiology-Legacy Content* 131, no. 3 (December 31, 1940): 639–49. https://doi.org/10.1152/ajplegacy.1940.131.3.639.

Roberto, Christina A., Peter D. Larsen, Henry Agnew, Jenny Baik, and Kelly D. Brownell. "Evaluating the Impact of Menu Labeling on Food Choices and Intake." *American Journal of Public Health* 100, no. 2 (February 2010): 312–18. https://doi.org/10.2105/AJPH.2009.160226.

Robinson, Mike J. F., Patrick Anselme, Adam M. Fischer, and Kent C. Berridge. "Initial Uncertainty in Pavlovian Reward Prediction Persistently Elevates Incentive Salience and Extends Sign-Tracking to Normally Unattractive Cues." *Behavioural Brain Research* 266 (June 2014): 119–30. https://doi.org/10.1016/j.bbr.2014.03.004.

Robinson, T. "The Neural Basis of Drug Craving: An Incentive-Sensitization Theory of Addiction." *Brain Research Reviews* 18, no. 3 (December 1993): 247–91. https://doi.org/10.1016/0165-0173(93)90013-P.

Rogers, P. J., P. S. Hogenkamp, C. de Graaf, S. Higgs, A. Lluch, A. R. Ness, C. Penfold, et al. "Does Low-Energy Sweetener Consumption Affect Energy Intake and Body Weight? A Systematic Review, Including Meta-Analyses, of the Evidence from Human and Animal Studies." *International Journal of Obesity* 40, no. 3 (March 2016): 381–94. https://doi.org/10.1038/ijo.2015.177.

Roig, M. G., Z. S. Rivera, and J. F. Kennedy. "A Model Study on Rate of Degradation of L-Ascorbic Acid during Processing Using Home-Produced Juice Concentrates." *International Journal of Food Sciences and Nutrition* 46, no. 2 (January 1995): 107–15. https://doi.org/10.3109/09637489509012538.

Roller, Sibel, and Sylvia A. Jones, eds. *Handbook of Fat Replacers*. Boca Raton, FL: CRC Press, 1996.

Rolls, B. J., P. A. Pirraglia, M. B. Jones, and J. C. Peters. "Effects of Olestra, a Noncaloric Fat Substitute, on Daily Energy and Fat Intakes in Lean

Men." *American Journal of Clinical Nutrition* 56, no. 1 (July 1, 1992): 84–92. https://doi.org/10.1093/ajcn/56.1.84.

Rolls, E. T. "The Neural Basis of Brain-Stimulation Reward." *Progress in Neurobiology* 3 (January 1974): 71–118. https://doi.org/10.1016/0301-0082(74)90005-7.

Rozin, Paul. "The Selection of Foods by Rats, Humans, and Other Animals." In *Advances in the Study of Behavior*, vol. 6, edited by Jay Rosenblatt, Robert Hinde, Evelyn Shaw, and Colin Beer, 21–76. Amsterdam: Academic Press, 1976. https://doi.org/10.1016/S0065-3454(08)60081-9.

Rudenga, K. J., and D. M. Small. "Amygdala Response to Sucrose Consumption Is Inversely Related to Artificial Sweetener Use." *Appetite* 58, no. 2 (April 2012): 504–7. https://doi.org/10.1016/j.appet.2011.12.001.

Safranski, Rüdiger, and David B. Dollenmayer. *Goethe: Life as a Work of Art.* New York: Liveright, 2017.

Sainsbury, A., and L. Zhang. "Role of the Hypothalamus in the Neuroendocrine Regulation of Body Weight and Composition during Energy Deficit: Endocrine Control of Body Composition." *Obesity Reviews* 13, no. 3 (March 2012): 234–57. https://doi.org/10.1111/j.1467-789X.2011.00948.x.

Salimpoor, Valorie N, Mitchel Benovoy, Kevin Larcher, Alain Dagher, and Robert J. Zatorre. "Anatomically Distinct Dopamine Release during Anticipation and Experience of Peak Emotion to Music." *Nature Neuroscience* 14, no. 2 (February 2011): 257–62. https://doi.org/10.1038/nn.2726.

Sanders, Tom, and Peter Emery. *Molecular Basis of Human Nutrition.* London and New York: Taylor and Francis, 2003.

Schultz, Wolfram, Kerstin Preuschoff, Colin Camerer, Ming Hsu, Christopher D Fiorillo, Philippe N. Tobler, and Peter Bossaerts. "Explicit Neural Signals Reflecting Reward Uncertainty." *Philosophical Transactions of the Royal Society B: Biological Sciences* 363, no. 1511 (December 12, 2008): 3801–11. https://doi.org/10.1098/rstb.2008.0152.

Seamon, David, and Arthur Zajonc, eds. *Goethe's Way of Science: A Phenomenology of Nature.* SUNY Series in Environmental and Architectural Phenomenology. Albany: State University of New York Press, 1998.

Sette, S., C. Le Donne, R. Piccinelli, D. Arcella, A. Turrini, and C. Leclercq. "The Third Italian National Food Consumption Survey, INRAN-SCAI 2005–06—Part 1: Nutrient Intakes in Italy." *Nutrition, Metabolism and Cardiovascular Diseases* 21, no. 12 (December 2011): 922–32. https://doi.org/10.1016/j.numecd.2010.03.001.

Shell, Ellen Ruppell. *The Hungry Gene: The Inside Story of the Obesity Industry.* New York: Grove Press, 2003.

Shepherd, Gordon M. *Neuroenology: How the Brain Creates the Taste of Wine.* New York: Columbia University Press, 2017.

———. *Neurogastronomy: How the Brain Creates Flavor and Why It Matters.* New York: Columbia University Press, 2012.

Small, D. M., R. J. Zatorre, A. Dagher, A. C. Evans, and M. Jones-Gotman. "Changes in Brain Activity Related to Eating Chocolate: From Pleasure to Aversion." *Brain: A Journal of Neurology* 124, pt. 9 (September 2001): 1720–33. https://doi.org/10.1093/brain/124.9.1720.

Smeets, Wilhelmus J. A. J. "Distribution of Dopamine Immunoreactivity in the Forebrain and Midbrain of the Snake *Python regius*: A Study with Antibodies against Dopamine." *Journal of Comparative Neurology* 271, no. 1 (May 1, 1988): 115–29. https://doi.org/10.1002/cne.902710112.

Stice, Eric, Sonja Spoor, Cara Bohon, Marga G. Veldhuizen, and Dana M. Small. "Relation of Reward from Food Intake and Anticipated Food Intake to Obesity: A Functional Magnetic Resonance Imaging Study." *Journal of Abnormal Psychology* 117, no. 4 (2008): 924–35. https://doi.org/10.1037/a0013600.

Stice, Eric, and Sonja Yokum. "Neural Vulnerability Factors That Increase Risk for Future Weight Gain." *Psychological Bulletin* 142, no. 5 (May 2016): 447–71. https://doi.org/10.1037/bul0000044.

Strausfeld, N. J., and F. Hirth. "Deep Homology of Arthropod Central Complex and Vertebrate Basal Ganglia." *Science* 340, no. 6129 (April 12, 2013): 157–61. https://doi.org/10.1126/science.1231828.

Swithers, Susan E., and Terry L. Davidson. "A Role for Sweet Taste: Calorie Predictive Relations in Energy Regulation by Rats." *Behavioral Neuroscience* 122, no. 1 (2008): 161–73. https://doi.org/10.1037/0735-7044.122.1.161.

Swithers, Susan E., Sean B. Ogden, and Terry L. Davidson. "Fat Substitutes Promote Weight Gain in Rats Consuming High-Fat Diets." *Behavioral Neuroscience* 125, no. 4 (2011): 512–18. https://doi.org/10.1037/a0024404.

Szeto, Ignatius M. Y., Alfred Aziz, Paul J. Das, Ameer Y. Taha, Nobuhiko Okubo, Sandra Reza-Lopez, Adria Giacca, and G. Harvey Anderson. "High Multivitamin Intake by Wistar Rats during Pregnancy Results in Increased Food Intake and Components of the Metabolic Syndrome in Male Offspring." *American Journal of Physiology-Regulatory, Integrative and Comparative Physiology* 295, no. 2 (August 2008): R575–82. https://doi.org/10.1152/ajpregu.90354.2008.

Taubes, Gary. "What If It's All Been a Big Fat Lie." *New York Times Magazine,* July 7, 2002.

Tchicaya, Anastase, and Nathalie Lorentz. "Socioeconomic Inequality and Obesity Prevalence Trends in Luxembourg, 1995–2007." *BMC Research Notes* 5, no. 1 (December 2012): 467. https://doi.org/10.1186/1756-0500-5-467.

Tellez, Luis A, Wenfei Han, Xiaobing Zhang, Tatiana L. Ferreira, Isaac O. Perez, Sara J. Shammah-Lagnado, Anthony N. van den Pol, and Ivan E. de Araujo. "Separate Circuitries Encode the Hedonic and Nutritional Values of Sugar." *Nature Neuroscience* 19, no. 3 (March 2016): 465–70. https://doi.org/10.1038/nn.4224.

Tellez, Luis A., Xueying Ren, Wenfei Han, Sara Medina, Jozélia G. Ferreira, Catherine W. Yeckel, and Ivan E. de Araujo. "Glucose Utilization Rates Regulate Intake Levels of Artificial Sweeteners: Glucose Utilization and Artificial Sweeteners." *Journal of Physiology* 591, no. 22 (November 15, 2013): 5727–44. https://doi.org/10.1113/jphysiol.2013.263103.

Todes, Daniel Philip. *Ivan Pavlov: A Russian Life in Science*. Oxford, UK: Oxford University Press, 2014.

Turrini, A., A. Saba, D. Perrone, E. Cialfa, and A. D'Amicis. "Food Consumption Patterns in Italy: The INN-CA Study 1994–1996." *European Journal of Clinical Nutrition* 55, no. 7 (July 2001): 571–88. https://doi.org/10.1038/sj.ejcn.1601185.

United States Census Bureau. "The 2012 Statistical Abstract. Health & Nutrition: Food Consumption and Nutrition. Table 217. Per Capita Consumption of Major Food Commodities: 1980 to 2009." United States Census Bureau, 2012.

United States Department of Agriculture. *Keeping Livestock Healthy: Yearbook of Agriculture 1942*. USDA, 1942.

Vandewater, Elizabeth A., Mi-suk Shim, and Allison G. Caplovitz. "Linking Obesity and Activity Level with Children's Television and Video Game Use." *Journal of Adolescence* 27, no. 1 (February 2004): 71–85. https://doi.org/10.1016/j.adolescence.2003.10.003.

Veldhuizen, Maria Geraldine, Richard Keith Babbs, Barkha Patel, Wambura Fobbs, Nils B. Kroemer, Elizabeth Garcia, Martin R. Yeomans, and Dana M. Small. "Integration of Sweet Taste and Metabolism Determines Carbohydrate Reward." *Current Biology* 27, no. 16 (August 2017): 2476–85.e6. https://doi.org/10.1016/j.cub.2017.07.018.

Wamala, Sarah P., Alicja Wolk, and Kristina Orth-Gomér. "Determinants of Obesity in Relation to Socioeconomic Status among Middle-Aged Swedish Women." *Preventive Medicine* 26, no. 5 (September 1997): 734–44. https://doi.org/10.1006/pmed.1997.0199.

Weise Prinzo, Zita. "Pellagra: And Its Prevention and Control in Major Emergencies." World Health Organization, 2000.

Weller, Rosalyn E., Edwin W. Cook, Kathy B. Avsar, and James E. Cox. "Obese
    Women Show Greater Delay Discounting than Healthy-Weight Women."
    Appetite 51, no. 3 (November 2008): 563–69. https://doi.org/10.1016/j.
    appet.2008.04.010.
Westerterp, Klaas R. *Energy Balance in Motion.* New York: SpringerLink, 2013.
Wheeler, G. A. "The Alleged Production of Pellagra by an Unbalanced Diet—
    A Reply." *Journal of the American Medical Association* 56, no. 13 (March 25,
    1916): 977. https://doi.org/10.1001/jama.1916.02580390047027.
Wilen, Richard, and Frederick Naftolin. "Pubertal Food Intake and Body
    Length, Weight, and Composition in the Feed-Restricted Female Rat:
    Comparison with Well Fed Animals." *Pediatric Research* 12, no. 4 (April
    1978): 263–67. https://doi.org/10.1203/00006450-197804000-00003.
Wise, Roy A. "Dopamine and Reward: The Anhedonia Hypothesis 30 Years
    On." *Neurotoxicity Research* 14, no. 2–3 (June 2008): 169–83. https://doi
    .org/10.1007/BF03033808.
———. "The Dopamine Synapse and the Notion of 'Pleasure Centers' in the
    Brain." *Trends in Neurosciences* 3, no. 4 (April 1980): 91–95. https://doi.
    org/10.1016/0166-2236(80)90035-1.
Wollenberg, R. A. C. "Pellagra in Italy." *Public Health Reports (1896–1970)* 24,
    no. 30 (1909): 1051. https://doi.org/10.2307/4563397.
Woods, Stephen C. "The Eating Paradox: How We Tolerate Food." *Psycho-
    logical Review* 98, no. 4 (1991): 488–505. https://doi.org/10.1037/0033
    -295X.98.4.488.
Yang, Hae Kyung, Kyungdo Han, Jae-Hyoung Cho, Kun-Ho Yoon, Bong-Yun
    Cha, and Seung-Hwan Lee. "Ambient Temperature and Prevalence of
    Obesity: A Nationwide Population-Based Study in Korea." Edited by
    David Meyre. *PLOS ONE* 10, no. 11 (November 2, 2015): e0141724.
    https://doi.org/10.1371/journal.pone.0141724.
Zhang, Guoxin, Zhentao Zhang, Ling Liu, Jiaolong Yang, Jinsha Huang, Nian
    Xiong, and Tao Wang. "Impulsive and Compulsive Behaviors in Parkin-
    son's Disease." *Frontiers in Aging Neuroscience* 6 (November 14, 2014).
    https://doi.org/10.3389/fnagi.2014.00318.
Zhu, Yong, Walter H. Hsu, and James H. Hollis. "Modified Sham Feeding of
    Foods with Different Macronutrient Compositions Differentially Influ-
    ences Cephalic Change of Insulin, Ghrelin, and NMR-Based Metabolo-
    mic Profiles." *Physiology & Behavior* 135 (August 2014): 135–42. https://
    doi.org/10.1016/j.physbeh.2014.06.009.

Notes

Introduction: The Mystery

1 *scientific feeding of carbohydrates:* Hall et al., "Energy Expenditure and Body Composition Changes after an Isocaloric Ketogenic Diet in Overweight and Obese Men."

3 *"What If It's All Been a Big Fat Lie":* Taubes, "What If It's All Been a Big Fat Lie."

4 *According to the "carbohydrate-insulin model":* Ludwig and Ebbeling, "The Carbohydrate-Insulin Model of Obesity"; and Hu et al., "The Carbohydrate-Insulin Model Does Not Explain the Impact of Varying Dietary Macronutrients on the Body Weight and Adiposity of Mice."

6 *another fat-carb study:* Gardner et al., "Effect of Low-Fat vs Low-Carbohydrate Diet on 12-Month Weight Loss in Overweight Adults and the Association With Genotype Pattern or Insulin Secretion."

7 *range of success:* Belluz, "Why Do Dieters Succeed or Fail? The Answers Have Little to Do with Food."

7 *dozens of controlled feeding experiments:* Hall and Guo, "Obesity Energetics." This 2017 meta-analysis of thirty-two controlled feeding studies found that when comparing both energy expenditure and fat loss, low-fat diets have a slight edge over low-carb diets. For a more recent study comparing ketogenic and low-fat diets: Buga et al., "The Effects of a 6-Week Controlled, Hypocaloric Ketogenic Diet, With and Without Exogenous Ketone Salts, on Body Composition Responses."

7 *It stayed even:* United States Census Bureau, "The 2012 Statistical Abstract. Health & Nutrition: Food Consumption and Nutrition. Table 217. Per Capita Consumption of Major Food Commodities: 1980 to 2009."

8 *About fifteen pounds per person:* According to the USDA Economic Research Service Food Availability Data System, from 2000 to 2019 American annual wheat availability fell from 146.3 lb./person to 131.1 lb./person.

8 *from forty-seven teaspoons per day to thirty-eight:* According to the USDA Economic Research Service

8 *obesity has climbed from:* According to the Centers for Disease Control.

8 *enormous, extremely expensive study:* Howard et al., "Low-Fat Dietary Pattern."

8 *never quite got the answer:* "As a result, differences in CVD risk factors between the intervention and comparison groups were minimal—e.g., at year 3, there were net reductions of 3.55 mg/dL in levels of low-density lipoprotein cholesterol and less than 1 mm Hg in blood pressure." Anderson and Appel, "Dietary Modification and CVD Prevention."

9 *an editorial in the* Journal of the American Medical Association: Ibid.

9 *a group of scientists at Yale University:* Roberto et al., "Evaluating the Impact of Menu Labeling."

9 *But it didn't last:* For more review of the generally disappointing effects of calorie counts, see Cantu-Jungles et al., "A Meta-Analysis to Determine the Impact of Restaurant Menu Labeling on Calories and Nutrients (Ordered or Consumed) in U.S. Adults."

9 *five years after the law was passed:* Cantor et al., "Five Years Later."

9 *the weight comes back:* Chow and Hall, "Short- and Long-Term Energy Intake Patterns and Their Implications for Human Body Weight Regulation."

9 *two-thirds will eventually regain:* Mann et al., "Medicare's Search for Effective Obesity Treatments."

9 *a life-consuming effort:* Personal correspondence with James Hill.

Part One: One Disease, Two Cures

Chapter 1. The New Road to Better Nutrition

15 *his creative output had stalled:* Safranski and Dollenmayer, *Goethe*, 271.

15 *odd brownish cast: The Works of J. W. von Goethe*, vol 12, *Letters from Italy*, pt. 2.

15 *rough skin:* Ginnaio, "La pellagre en Italie, à la fin du XIXe siècle : les effets d'une maladie de carence," Ibid., 585.

16 *set off wandering:* Ibid., 589.

16 *threw it out the window:* Cesar Ruggieri, MD, "Narrative of the Crucifixion of Mattio Lovat," *The Pamphleteer*, May 1814, 363–64. "As his age

increased, he became subject in the spring to giddiness in his head, and eruptions of a leprous appearance showed themselves on his face and hands. . . . These are the symptoms of that cruel malady, the existence of which in several of our provinces, is but too well confirmed by the ravages which it has made in them."

16 *Other theories ran the gamut:* Ginnaio, "La pellagre en Italie à la fin du XIXe siècle : les effets d'une maladie de carence"; and McDowell, *Vitamin History.*

17 *more than 104,000 Italians:* Wollenberg, "Pellagra in Italy," 1051–54.

17 *Pellagra had come to the United States:* Rajakumar, "Pellagra in the United States."

17 *By 1906:* Bollet, "Politics and Pellagra."

17 *within two years:* Deaderick, William, and Loyd Thompson, "The Endemic Diseases of the Southern States," *Journal of the American Medical Association* 67, no. 7, 1916, p. 285.

17 *relation to water:* Ibid.

17 *Mount Vernon Hospital for the Colored Insane:* Rajakumar, "Pellagra in the United States."

18 *More experiments were conducted:* Deaderick and Thompson "Endemic Diseases of the Southern States."

18 *carried by insects:* Ibid., 306.

18 *a Hungarian-born Jew:* Rajakumar, "Pellagra in the United States."

18 *172 children had been diagnosed:* Ibid.

18 *Goldberger explicitly instructed staff:* Morabia, "Joseph Goldberger's Research on the Prevention of Pellagra."

19 *a dietary disorder:* Goldberger, Wariu, and Willets, "The Prevention of Pellagra. A test of Diet Among Institutional Inmates."

19 *"half baked":* Kraut, Alan, "Dr. Joseph Goldberger. & the War on Pellagra," The Office of NIH History & Stetten Museum, National Institutes of Health, https://history.nih.gov/pages/viewpage.action?pageId=8883184

19 *a long and bizarre article:* Wheeler, "The Alleged Production of Pellagra by an Unbalanced Diet—A Reply."

19 *"filth parties":* Kraut, Alan, "Dr. Joseph Goldberger & the War on Pellagra,"; The Office of NIH History & Stetten Museum, National Institutes of Health, https://history.nih.gov/pages/viewpage.action?pageId=8883184; and Bollet, "Politics and Pellagra."

19 *He extracted:* Goldberger, "Public Health Reports."

19 *"from fence post to fence post":* Otto, *The Final Frontiers, 1880-1930.* 72.

20 *Pellagra Squad:* "Goldberger: An Unremitting Struggle to Conquer Pellagra."

20 *owned by their landlord:* Ibid.; and *The Final Frontiers, 1880-1930: Settling the Southern Bottomlands*, 72, and DeKleine, "Recent Trends in Pellagra."

20 *nourish your infant:* Ginnaio, "La pellagre en Italie. à la fin du XIXe siècle: les effets d'une maladie de carence"

20 *killed more than one hundred thousand Americans:* Marks, "Epidemiologists Explain Pellagra."

20 *In the spring of 1927:* Kruif, *The Fight for Life*, 15.

21 *was fed to dogs sick with pellagra:* Elvehjem et al., "Relation of Nicotinic Acid and Nicotinic Acid Amide to Canine Black Tongue."

21 *a glow of health swept over them:* Rachmilewitz and Glueck, "Treatment of Pellagra with Nicotinic Acid."

21 *the US government decided:* Bishai and Nalubola, "The History of Food Fortification in the United States."

22 *the law of the land:* "Effectiveness of Food Fortification, in the United States." 733.

22 *in a single year:* Ibid., 736.

23 *pellagra did in forty:* Obesity is annually responsible for at least 325,000 unnecessary deaths in the United States, whereas from 1906 to 1940, the pellagra epidemic is believed to have killed 100,000 Americans. Allison, "Annual Deaths Attributable to Obesity in the United States"; and Bollet, "Politics and Pellagra."

23 *television:* Dietz and Gortmaker, "Do We Fatten Our Children at the Television Set?"

23 *cars:* Frank, Andresen, and Schmid, "Obesity Relationships with Community Design, Physical Activity, and Time Spent in Cars."

23 *escalators:* Meyers et al., "Stairs, Escalators, and Obesity."

23 *video games:* Vandewater, Shim, and Caplovitz, "Linking Obesity and Activity Level with Children's Television and Video Game Use."

23 *supermarkets:* Kimenju et al., "Do Supermarkets Contribute to the Obesity Pandemic in Developing Countries?"

23 *a lack of supermarkets:* Morland, Diez Roux, and Wing, "Supermarkets, Other Food Stores, and Obesity."

23 *artificial lighting:* Park et al., "Association of Exposure to Artificial Light at Night While Sleeping With Risk of Obesity in Women."

23 *air-conditioning:* Yang et al., "Ambient Temperature and Prevalence of Obesity."

Chapter 2. The Old Italian Way

25 *Italy's response to pellagra:* Ginnaio, "La pellagre en Italie à la fin du XIXe siècle: les effets d'une maladie de carence."

25 *Even wine:* Lee, *Observations on the Principal Medical Institutions & Practice of France, Italy, & Germany: With Notices of the Universities and Cases from Hospital Practice.*

25 *73,000 cases of pellagra:* Wollenberg, "Pellagra in Italy."

26 *Just 202 cases:* Ginnaio, "La pellagre en Italie à la fin du XIXe siècle: les effets d'une maladie de carence."

26 *The rate of obesity in Mississipi is 37 percent:* This figure seems at odds with a national rate of 42.4 percent because the former comes from the Behavioral Risk Factor Surveillance System and the latter from the National Health and Nutrition Examination Survey.

26 *by several pounds:* Comparing cheese consumption between a region of Italy and the entire United States is challenging since the figures for each region are derived using different measurements. That said, most assessments of national cheese consumption place Italy ahead of the United States, and surveys of Italians consumption, such as Turrini et al., "Food Consumption Patterns in Italy: The INN-CA Study 1994 ± 1996," indicated northerners consume significantly more cheese than southerners. Turrini et al., "Food Consumption Patterns in Italy."

28 *sausage wrapped in beef:* The dish is called *cotechino fasciato.*

29 *attracts nearly one foreign tourist:* According to "Travel & Tourism Economic Impact 2017 Italy," published by the World Travel & Tourism Council, Italy attracted 54.5 million tourists in 2016, as compared to an Italian population of 60.6 million.

29 *four times the US rate:* The United States attracts approximately 79 million tourists, according to the National Trade and Tourism Office.

29 *conducted a survey:* Personal correspondence with Erik Wolf, executive director, World Food Travel Association.

29 *Italian women:* Finucane et al., "Global Trends in Body-Mass Index since 1980," 563.

29 *decreased by thirty thousand:* Lauria et al., "Decline of Childhood Overweight and Obesity in Italy from 2008 to 2016." Childhood obesity in Italy is an enigma. The country has long had what appears to be elevated rates of childhood obesity, and yet it seems to disappear in adult cohorts.

30 *American woman gained around twenty pounds:* According to the CDC, the average American woman weighed 145.4 pounds in 1976–80 and 166 pounds in 2007–8.

30 *In northern Italy:* US statistics are from the CDC. Italian statistics are taken from Gallus et al., "Overweight and Obesity Prevalence and Determinants in Italy: An Update to 2010." According to the study's lead author,

Silvano Gallus, the statistics are in broad agreement with the more recent study Gallus et al., "Overweight and Obesity in 16 European Countries."

31 *change in Italian eating:* Simona Giampaoli et al., "Comportamenti alimentari degli italiani: Risultati dell'osservatorio epidemiologico cardiovascolare / health examination survey," https://www.epiprev.it/materiali/2015/EP5-6/EP5-6_373_art14.pdf.

31 *migrate to America:* Danubio, Amicone, and Vargiu, "Height and BMI of Italian Immigrants to the USA, 1908–1970."

31 *Australia:* Astell-Burt et al., "Influence of Neighbourhood Ethnic Density, Diet and Physical Activity on Ethnic Differences in Weight Status."

31 *Switzerland:* Marques-Vidal et al., "Prevalence of Overweight and Obesity among Migrants in Switzerland."

32 *a third as much of soft drink:* According to Statista, Italians consumed 50 liters per capita in 2015, while Americans consumed 148 liters (39 gallons) per capita in 2018.

32 *more fish and less meat:* According to Giovanni De Gaetano, MD, PhD, head, Department of Epidemiology and Prevention, IRCCS Istituto Neurologico Mediterraneo (Neuromed), "In our late study from the INHES cohort (a 3-year telephone-based survey on nutrition and health, which, between November 2010 and November 2013, has recruited 9,319 women and men aged equal to or greater than 5 years from all over Italy) we have recently confirmed that people from the Southern regions are more likely to follow a Mediterranean diet as compared to the Northern area. Yet, southern adult (aged greater than18 years) individuals show higher prevalence of obesity."

32 *suffer from more heart disease:* Personal communication with Giovanni De Gaetano, MD, PhD, head, Department of Epidemiology and Prevention, IRCCS Istituto Neurologico Mediterraneo (Neuromed), who was referring to Progetto Cuore, a national population registry for monitoring cardiovascular disease and risk factors within the Italian adult population.

32 *northern Italian divorcées:* Gallus et al., "Overweight and Obesity Prevalence and Determinants in Italy."

Part II: You Are a Metabolic Genius (and You Love It)

Chapter 3. You're Hot. Then You're Not

37 *rinsed the bathtub:* Cabanac, *The Quest for Pleasure,* 19.

43 *7,945 calories:* Cabanac, Duclaux, and Spector, "Sensory Feedback in Regulation of Body Weight."

45 *weight loss hits a plateau:* Polidori et al., "How Strongly Does Appetite Counter Weight Loss?," 2293.

45 *a physician named Jules Hirsch discovered:* Kolata, *Rethinking Thin*, 113.

46 *profound physiological changes:* https://www.dana.org/article/obesity -matter-over-mind/; and Kolata, *Rethinking Thin*.

46 *people who were starving:* Details of Minnesota Starvation Experiment taken from Kolata, *Rethinking Thin*; and Kalm and Semba, "They Starved So That Others Be Better Fed."

47 *were experiencing starvation:* http://www.dana.org/Cerebrum/2003/ Obesity__Matter_Over_Mind_/.

47 *sensors in leg bones:* Jansson et al., "Body Weight Homeostat That Regulates Fat Mass Independently of Leptin in Rats and Mice."

47 *when they reach a certain weight:* Wilen and Naftolin, "Pubertal Food Intake and Body Length, Weight, and Composition in the Feed-Restricted Female Rat"; and Bratke et al., "Timing of Menarche in Norwegian Girls."

47 *these cells turn on:* Sainsbury and Zhang, "Role of the Hypothalamus in the Neuroendocrine Regulation of Body Weight and Composition during Energy Deficit."

47 *These cells are* turned off: Baskin, Hahn, and Schwartz, "Leptin Sensitive Neurons in the Hypothalamus."

47 *is almost never the same:* Edholm et al., "Food Intake and Energy Expenditure of Army Recruits."

47 *five times higher:* Westerterp and SpringerLink, *Energy Balance in Motion*, 67.

47 *scientists began tracking:* Kim et al., "Evaluation of Long-Term Dietary Intakes of Adults Consuming Self-Selected Diets."

47 *One woman's daily food diaries:* Data supplied by Kevin Hall.

48 *It followed:* Polidori et al., "How Strongly Does Appetite Counter Weight Loss?"

49 *studying the contestants:* Kerns et al., "Increased Physical Activity Associated with Less Weight Regain Six Years After 'The Biggest Loser' Competition."

49 *a follow-up study:* Fothergill et al., "Persistent Metabolic Adaptation 6 Years after 'The Biggest Loser' Competition."

50 *his weight remained oddly stable:* Bray, "Luxuskonsumption—Myth or Reality?"

50 *attempted to fatten his lab mice:* Kolata, *Rethinking Thin*, 116–18.

51 *drop out of the study:* Shell, *The Hungry Gene: The Inside Story of the Obesity Industry*, 80.

51 *one of the more unusual experiments:* Leibel, Rosenbaum, and Hirsch, "Changes in Energy Expenditure Resulting from Altered Body Weight."

52 *achieve a bulging stomach:* Garine and Koppert, "Guru-Fattening Sessions among The Massa."

53 *they are back where they started:* Pasquet and Apfelbaum, "Recovery of Initial Body Weight and Composition after Long-Term Massive Overfeeding in Men."

Chapter 4. The Quest for Pleasure

56 *"Cross-Cultural Differences in Simple Taste Preferences":* Moskowitz et al., "Cross-Cultural Differences in Simple Taste Preferences."

57 *Some tamarind is sweet:* Tamarind concentrations taken from El-Siddig, *Tamarind*, 16.

58 *is called jowar:* Basavaraja et al., "Kharif Sorghum in Karnataka: An Economic Analysis."

58 *the disease has been known:* Sanders and Emery, *Molecular Basis of Human Nutrition*, 122.

58 *three times as much niacin:* Indian tamarind contains a niacin equivalent of 2.24 mg/100 g, according to Frida Food Data, published by the National Food Institute, Technical University of Denmark, whereas milk contains a niacin equivalent of 0.8 mg/100 g according to Caballero, Finglas, and Toldrá, *Encyclopedia of Food and Health*.

59 *exacerbates fluoride's toxic effects:* Chandrashekar, Thankappan, and Sundaram, "Severe Dental Fluorosis and Jowar Consumption in Karnataka, India."

59 *experimental feedings of fluoride and tamarind:* Khandare, Uday Kumar, and Lakshmaiah, "Beneficial Effect of Tamarind Ingestion on Fluoride Toxicity in Dogs."

59 *a rural mystery:* Choubisa et al., "Food, Fluoride, and Fluorosis in Domestic Ruminants in the Dungarpur District of Rajasthan, India"; and Choubisa, "Natural Amelioration of Fluoride Toxicity (Fluorosis) in Goats and Sheep."

60 *protected them from fluoride toxicity:* Choubisa, "Natural Amelioration of Fluoride Toxicity (Fluorosis) in Goats and Sheep."

60 *Khandare began testing tamarind on humans:* Khandare et al., "Additional Beneficial Effect of Tamarind Ingestion over Defluoridated Water Supply to Adolescent Boys in a Fluorotic Area." See also Khandare, Rao, and Lakshmaiah, "Effect of Tamarind Ingestion on Fluoride Excretion in Humans."

60 *appeared to help remove fluoride:* Khandare et al., "Additional Beneficial Effect of Tamarind Ingestion over Defluoridated Water Supply to Adolescent Boys in a Fluorotic Area."

60 *Khandare visited a village:* Khandare et al., "Effects of Smoking, Use of Aluminium Utensils, and Tamarind Consumption on Fluorosis in a Fluorotic Village of Andhra Pradesh, India."

61 *"fluoride entrapment capacity":* Maruthamuthu and Reddy, "Binding of Fluoride with Tamarind Gel."

64 *"pleasure center":* Dror, "Cold War 'Super-Pleasure.'"

64 *The plan was as follows:* Olds, "Pleasure Centers in the Brain."

65 *self-stimulated more than 850,000 times:* Facts in this paragraph taken from Dror, "Cold War 'Super-Pleasure'"; and Rolls, "The Neural Basis of Brain-Stimulation Reward," 236.

66 *Grainy footage: The Mind,* documentary television episode featuring Robert Heath. Date and production details unknown.

66 *strangest and saddest experiments:* Moan and Heath, "Septal Stimulation for the Initiation of Heterosexual Behavior in a Homosexual Male."

67 *Your core is coolest at night:* Susanne La Fleur, personal communication.

Chapter 5. Too Much of a Good Thing

69 *Without dopamine, self-stimulation:* Wise, "Dopamine and Reward," 4.

70 *"pleasure, euphoria or yumminess":* Wise, "The Dopamine Synapse and the Notion of 'Pleasure Centers' in the Brain."

71 *eating triple the normal amount:* Berridge et al., "The Tempted Brain Eats," 6.

72 *they would do the strangest things:* Evans et al., "Punding in Parkinson's Disease."

72 *Elevated dopamine caused patients:* Politis et al., "Neural Response to Visual Sexual Cues in Dopamine Treatment-Linked Hypersexuality in Parkinson's Disease."

72 *slot machines and scratch cards:* Zhang et al., "Impulsive and Compulsive Behaviors in Parkinson's Disease."

72 *Others would pester their wives:* Berridge and Kringelbach, "Pleasure Systems in the Brain."

72 *derived no enjoyment:* Ibid.

72 *to go bowling:* Ibid.

73 *One study, from 1963:* Heath, "Electrical Self-Stimulation of the Brain in Man."

73 *went back to the case of B-19:* Berridge and Kringelbach, "Pleasure Systems in the Brain."

74 *if you flash an image:* Childress et al., "Prelude to Passion."

76 *yet are not addictive:* Robinson, "The Neural Basis of Drug Craving," 251.

78 *dismissing the very idea:* Berridge, " 'Liking' and 'Wanting' Food Rewards."

78 *overcome with anticipation:* Davis et al., "Dopamine for 'Wanting' and Opioids for 'Liking.' "

78 *adolescent girls with obesity experienced:* Stice et al., "Relation of Reward from Food Intake and Anticipated Food Intake to Obesity."

78 *went on to gain more weight:* Demos, Heatherton, and Kelley, "Individual Differences in Nucleus Accumbens Activity to Food and Sexual Images Predict Weight Gain and Sexual Behavior."

78 *months in the future:* Stice and Yokum, "Neural Vulnerability Factors That Increase Risk for Future Weight Gain."

Part III: Nutritive Mismatch

Chapter 6. How Sweet It Is

83 *most famous experiments:* Small et al., "Changes in Brain Activity Related to Eating Chocolate."

85 *The mice were put in cages with three sippers:* Araujo et al., "Food Reward in the Absence of Taste Receptor Signaling"; and Ren et al., "Nutrient Selection in the Absence of Taste Receptor Signaling."

85 *measured the exact patch of mouse brain:* Ferreira et al., "Regulation of Fat Intake in the Absence of Flavour Signalling."

85 *one that was even stranger:* Tellez et al., "Separate Circuitries Encode the Hedonic and Nutritional Values of Sugar."

86 *another mind-bending experiment:* Tellez et al., "Glucose Utilization Rates Regulate Intake Levels of Artificial Sweeteners."

87 *Small created five separate drinks:* Veldhuizen et al., "Integration of Sweet Taste and Metabolism Determines Carbohydrate Reward."

88 *To answer that question:* Ibid.

90 *a hallmark of diabetes called insulin sensitivity:* Dalenberg et al., "Short-Term Consumption of Sucralose with, but Not Without, Carbohydrate Impairs Neural and Metabolic Sensitivity to Sugar in Humans."

93 *Four entirely separate:* Personal correspondence, Alessia Ranciaro.

93 *as Daniel Nettle . . . has argued:* Nettle, Andrews, and Bateson, "Food Insecurity as a Driver of Obesity in Humans."

94 *"forces and loads":* Ibid.

94 *We stockpiled grain:* Kuijt and Finlayson, "Evidence for Food Storage and Predomestication Granaries 11,000 Years Ago in the Jordan Valley."

94 *smashed bison bones into pieces:* Personal correspondence with Trevor Peck.

95 *"I will eat this later":* Ibid.; and Peck, *Light from Ancient Campfires*; and personal correspondence with Trevor Peck.

95 *more DNA is devoted:* Shepherd, *Neurogastronomy,* 58.

95 *engages more gray matter:* Ibid., 13; Shepherd, *Neuroenology.*

Chapter 7. Not Losing Isn't Everything. It's the Only Thing

 99 *a jackpot totaling $39.7 million: Casino Life,* https://www.casinolifemagazine.com/article/biggest-slot-machine-wins-history.

100 *the Russian scientist observed that:* Todes, *Ivan Pavlov.*

101 *sold them as medications:* Ibid., 172.

101 *motivating effect:* Robinson et al., "Initial Uncertainty in Pavlovian Reward Prediction Persistently Elevates Incentive Salience and Extends Sign-Tracking to Normally Unattractive Cues."

102 *began studying the Pavlovian responses:* Brown and Jenkins, "Auto-Shaping of the Pigeon's Key-Peck."

102 *repeated the McMaster experiment:* Boakes, RA. "Performance on Learning to Associate a stimulus with positive rein- forcement."

103 *Around about the same time:* Kahneman and Teversky began their inquiry into decision theory five years before their paper on prospect theory was published, in 1979, and two years after the publication of Robert Boakes's paper on sign tracking and goal tracking.

103 *people gambled for a simple reason:* Anselme and Robinson, "What Motivates Gambling Behavior?"

103 *Here is an example:* Kahneman, *Thinking, Fast and Slow,* 280.

104 *another Kahneman-and-Tversky classic:* Kahneman and Tversky, "Prospect Theory," 266.

107 *a bitter pill to swallow:* Ibid., 286.

107 *who has not made peace:* Ibid., 287.

107 *Wolfram Schultz published the results:* Fiorillo, Tobler, and Schultz, "Discrete Coding of Reward Probability and Uncertainty by Dopamine Neurons." See also Schultz et al., "Explicit Neural Signals Reflecting Reward Uncertainty."

110 *A scientist at the University of Stockholm:* Forkman, "The Effect of Uncertainty on the Food Intake of the Mongolian Gerbil."

111 *took more time and effort:* Ibid.

113 *A study done in King County:* Drewnowski et al., "A New Method to Visualize Obesity Prevalence in Seattle-King County at the Census Block Level."

113 *The three poorest states:* The relative wealth of states here is measured according to median income.

113 *highest rates of obesity:* According to CDC 2019 Adult Obesity Prevalance Maps.

113 *Luxembourg:* Tchicaya and Lorentz, "Socioeconomic Inequality and Obesity Prevalence Trends in Luxembourg, 1995–2007."

113 *Australia:* O'Dea and Dibley, "Obesity Increase among Low SES Australian Schoolchildren between 2000 and 2006."

113 *Sweden:* Wamala, Wolk, and Orth-Gomér, "Determinants of Obesity in Relation to Socioeconomic Status among Middle-Aged Swedish Women."

113 *France:* Lioret et al., "Child Overweight in France and Its Relationship with Physical Activity, Sedentary Behaviour and Socioeconomic Status."

113 *England:* Booth, Charlton, and Gulliford, "Socioeconomic Inequality in Morbid Obesity with Body Mass Index More than 40 Kg/M2 in the United States and England."

113 *Scientists in Singapore:* Lim, Forde, and Cheon, "Low Subjective Socioeconomic Status Alters Taste-Based Perceptual Sensitivity to the Energy Density of Beverages."

113 *measured "food insecurity":* Nettle, Andrews, and Bateson, "Food Insecurity as a Driver of Obesity in Humans."

113 *the insurance hypothesis of obesity:* Ibid.

114 *they lunge for it:* Fisher and Birch, "Restricting Access to Palatable Foods Affects Children's Behavioral Response, Food Selection, and Intake."

114 *Mothers who tick:* Boots, Tiggemann, and Corsini, "Eating in the Absence of Hunger in Young Children."

Chapter 8. Creamfibre 7000

117 *"alginate ice-cream stabilizing composition":* US Patent 2485934.

118 *stretches back hundreds of millions of years:* Personal correspondence with Danielle Reed and Paul Breslin.

119 *presented this very condition:* Swithers and Davidson, "A Role for Sweet Taste."

120 *a tiny amount of weight:* Azad et al., "Nonnutritive Sweeteners and Cardiometabolic Health."

120 *studied it for clues:* Rogers et al., "Does Low-Energy Sweetener Consumption Affect Energy Intake and Body Weight?"

121 *"reward value":* Green and Murphy, "Altered Processing of Sweet Taste in the Brain of Diet Soda Drinkers"; and Rudenga and Small, "Amygdala Re-

sponse to Sucrose Consumption Is Inversely Related to Artificial Sweetener Use."

121 *eliminating these faults:* Personal correspondence with Kathryn Deibler.

122 *three hundred and sixty-five thousand tons:* According to Industry Experts, Inc.

122 *did an olestra version:* Swithers, Ogden, and Davidson, "Fat Substitutes Promote Weight Gain in Rats Consuming High-Fat Diets."

123 *back in 1992:* Rolls et al., "Effects of Olestra, a Noncaloric Fat Substitute, on Daily Energy and Fat Intakes in Lean Men."

123 *America ate more fat replacers:* Fat replacer statistics courtesy of Markets andMarkets.

124 *all of ten cents:* According to MarketsandMarkets (personal correspondence), a carbohydrate-based fat replacer costs about $3.50 per kilogram. A 30-gram portion making up 20 percent of a 150-gram serving of low-fat yogurt would cost about ten cents at thirty-five cents per 100 grams.

125 *discovered in 1979:* Coy, "Discovery of Simplesse Was an Accident."

125 *40–50 billion:* Haddix, "That Phenomenon Simplesse Supplies the Feeling of Fat."

125 *"fat replacement in muffins":* Ceamfibre by CEAMSA for Bakery Applications.

126 *as if it came from a farm:* Simplesse brochure, CP Kelco. Similar descriptions in this paragraph are taken from corporate brochures.

126 *"combination systems":* Roller and Jones, *Handbook of Fat Replacers*, 18.

127 *dreadful puddles of water:* Corriher, "Science of Starch for the Perfect Sauce."

127 *created in 1967:* BeMiller, "One Hundred Years of Commercial Food Carbohydrates in the United States."

130 *spend less than half as much time eating:* http://www.oecd.org/gender /balancing-paid-work-unpaid-work-and-leisure.htm.

Part IV: The Help That Hurts

Chapter 9. Why Does Food Taste Good, Anyway?

133 *"My lust to see this land":* Safranski and Dollenmayer, *Goethe.*

134 *"and devoured the inner part":* This, along with many other details of Goethe's journey to Italy, are taken from *The Works of J. W. von Goethe*, vol. 12, *Letters from Italy*, pt. 2.

134 *slim and tanned:* Safranski and Dollenmayer, *Goethe*, 297.

135 *he seemed newly "sensual":* Ibid., 299.

135 *managed to procure foie gras:* http://goethetc.blogspot.com/2009/08/goethe
-as-gourmand.html.

135 *copycat suicides:* Furedi, "The Media's First Moral Panic."

136 *laughing it up with guests:* Safranski and Dollenmayer, *Goethe*, 211.

138 *a close match to our own:* Smeets, "Distribution of Dopamine Immunoreactivity in the Forebrain and Midbrain of the SnakePython Regius"; and
personal correspondence with Kurth Schwenk.

138 *600 million years ago:* Strausfeld and Hirth, "Deep Homology of Arthropod Central Complex and Vertebrate Basal Ganglia."

139 *almost never poisonous:* Some snakes, such as garter snakes, can secrete
ingested toxins through their skin.

139 *sight or aroma:* Woods, "The Eating Paradox."

139 *festival of gastric secretion:* Zhu, Hsu, and Hollis, "Modified Sham Feeding
of Foods with Different Macronutrient Compositions Differentially Influences Cephalic Change of Insulin, Ghrelin, and NMR-Based Metabolo-
mic Profiles."

139 *temporary case of diabetes:* Woods, "The Eating Paradox: How We Tolerate Food," 492.

140 *miraculous case of Tom:* "Human Gastric Function."

141 *the same "reward centers":* Gebauer, Kringelbach, and Vuust, "Ever-
Changing Cycles" of Musical Pleasure"; and Salimpoor et al., "Anatomi-
cally Distinct Dopamine Release during Anticipation and Experience of
Peak Emotion to Music."

142 *"violate" expectations:* Gebauer, Kringelbach, and Vuust, "Ever-Changing
Cycles. of Musical Pleasure"

143 *carnivores such as sea lions:* Jiang et al., "Major Taste Loss in Carnivorous
Mammals."

144 *goats of Olympic National Park:* "Mountain Goat Capture and Translo-
cation," National Park Service, https://www.nps.gov/olym/planyourvisit/
mountain-goat-capture-and-translocation.htm; and Blum, "Mountain
Goats Are Being Airlifted Out of a National Park Because They Crave
Human Pee."

144 *vitamins become scarce:* Barnes et al., "Prevention of Coprophagy in the
Rat."

145 *In the year 1602:* This and other anecdotes of scurvy and its effect on the
appetite taken from Carpenter, *The History of Scurvy and Vitamin C.*

146 *protects vitamin C from breaking down:* Roig, Rivera, and Kennedy, "A
Model Study on Rate of Degradation of L-Ascorbic Acid during Processing Using Home-Produced Juice Concentrates."

146 *"depraved appetites"*: Fleissner, "Earth-Eating, Addiction, Nostalgia: Charles Chesnutt's Diasporic Regionalism."

146 *"actually a kind of remedy"*: Mason, "On Atrophia a Ventriculo (Mal d'Estomac) or Dirt-Eating."

147 *"a clear marker of risk"*: Miao, Young, and Golden, "Meta-Analysis of Pica and Micronutrient Status."

147 *"invincible craving"*: Fleissner, "Earth-Eating, Addiction, Nostalgia: Charles Chesnutt's Diasporic Regionalism."

148 *"never wish to forget the brutal rapture"*: Ibid., 170.

Chapter 10, You Are Eating Pig Feed

150 *effectively become law:* Enrichment is not a federal law. However, since the majority of states mandate the enrichment of flour, it is effectively a national policy because millers do not wish to produce products that are not permitted for sale in certain states. According to the Food Fortification Initiative, 91 percent of wheat flour in the United States is fortified.

150 *in the early 1940s:* USDA Economic Research Service.

152 *"inadequate for optimum growth"*: McMillen, Luecke, and Thorp, "The Effect of Liberal B-Vitamin Supplementation on Growth of Weanling Pigs Fed Rations Containing a Variety of Feedstuffs."

152 *1942 Yearbook of Agriculture:* US Department of Agriculture, *Keeping Livestock Health*y: Yearbook of Agriculture 1942, 810.

152 *the experiment at the University of Illinois:* Dyer, Krider, and Carroll, "Known and Unidentified Factors Supplement a Corn-Soybean Meal Ration for Weanling Pigs in Drylot." See also McMillen, Luecke, and Thorp, "The Effect of Liberal B-Vitamin Supplementation on Growth of Weanling Pigs Fed Rations Containing a Variety of Feedstuffs."

153 *another grand experiment:* Hutchinson et al., "Comparison of Free-Choice and Complete Rations for Growing-Finishing Pigs on Pasture and Drylot."

155 *In 1959, the University of Illinois:* D. E. Becker, "Balancing Swine Rations," Circular 811, University of Illinois College of Agriculture Extension Service in Agriculture and Home Economics.

156 *fed up to four times as much niacin:* Ibid., for 1950s vitamin requirements and recommended fortification taken from "Balancing Swine Rations. The National Research Council's *Nutrient Requirements of Swine* (2012) reports a niacin requirement for pigs at all weights of 30 mg/kg (14 mg/lb). The Pork Information Gateway (US Pork Center of Excellence) reports additions of niacin at up to 25 mg/lb and riboflavin at 10 mg/lb, as compared to 7.5 mg/lb and 0.5 mg/lb recommended fortification in "Bal-

ancing Swine Rations." Real et al., "Effects of Increasing Dietary Niacin, on Growth Performance and Meat Quality in Finishing Pigs Reared in Two Different Environments1,2" found that pigs fed a basal diet of corn and soybean require up to 55 mg/kg of added niacin to maximize daily gain and feed efficiency.

158 *the rat moms:* Pannia et al., "High Multivitamin Diet Fed to Wistar Rat Dams during Pregnancy Increases Maternal Weight Gain Later in Life and Alters Homeostatic, Hedonic and Peripheral Regulatory Systems of Energy Balance."

158 *preordained for a lifetime of weight gain:* Szeto et al., "High Multivitamin Intake by Wistar Rats during Pregnancy Results in Increased Food Intake and Components of the Metabolic Syndrome in Male Offspring"; and Reza-López et al., "High Vitamin Intake by Wistar Rats during Pregnancy Alters Tissue Fatty Acid Concentration in the Offspring Fed an Obe-sogenic Diet."

158 *"plays a central role in":* These generic descriptions of vitamin action are taken from Wikipedia.

159 *consumed about 1.4 milligrams:* According to the USDA Economic Re-search Service.

160 *550-pound man:* This is an estimate. According to Institute of Medicine (US), *Dietary Reference Intakes for Thiamin, Riboflavin, Niacin, Vitamin B_6, Folate, Vitamin B_{12}, Pantothenic Acid, Biotin, and Choline,* the esti-mated average requirement for thiamin is 0.3 mg per 1,000 kcal. Thus 3 mg of thiamin is an order of magnitude higher, which is enough thiamin for a diet of 10,000 kcal per day. If we use the NIH Body Weight Planner, even a physically active man would need to weigh in excess of 250 kg to maintain such a diet. Institute of Medicine (U.S.), Institute of Medicine (U.S.), and Institute of Medicine (U.S.), *Dietary Reference Intakes for Thi-amin, Riboflavin, Niacin, Vitamin B,ÇÜ, Folate, Vitamin B,ÇÅ,ÇÇ, Panto-thenic Acid, Biotin, and Choline.*

160 *ingestion of thiamin chloride:* Richter and Hawkes, "The Dependence of the Carbohydrate, Fat and Protein Appetite of Rats on the Various Com-ponents of the Vitamin B Complex."

160 *unusual relationship with niacin:* Hundley, "Influence of Fructose and Other Carbohydrates on the Niacin Requirement of the Rat."

160 *105 pounds of sugar and high fructose corn syrup:* According to the USDA Economic Research Service.

161 *more than triple the required amount:* This figure is based on the 1993 "Re-port of the Nova Scotia Nutrition Survey," as well as the "Les Québécoises et les Québécois Mangent-Ils Mieux? Rapport de l'Enquête Québécoise

sur la Nutrition," 1990, both of which measure niacin equivalent intake, which includes the conversion of tryptophan to niacin. In each case, average consumption is more than triple the estimated average requirement. Canadian intakes, furthermore, are likely lower than American intakes. https://www.ncbi.nlm.nih.gov/books/NBK114320/; and https://www.ncbi.nlm.nih.gov/books/NBK114304/.

161 *triple that amount yet again:* https://ods.od.nih.gov/factsheets/Niacin-HealthProfessional/#h4.

161 *a single milligram of thiamin per day:* Sette et al., "The Third Italian National Food Consumption Survey, INRAN-SCAI 2005–06–Part 1."

161 *less than what Americans consumed in 1940:* Calculated by USDA / Center for Nutrition Policy and Promotion.

162 *half as much niacin and riboflavin:* Riboflavin consumption taken from Sette et al., "The third Italian National Food Consumption Survey"; INRAN-SCAI 2005e06 e Part 1: Nutrient intakes in Italy" and "Vitamins Pper Capita per Day in the U.S. Food Supply, 1909–2010. 1"; Niacin comparison is made with niacin equivalent, which includes conversion of tryptophan. Italian data taken from "Tolerable Upper Intake Levels for Vitamins and Minerals"; and US data is inferred from "Report of the Nova Scotia Nutrition Survey," as well as the "Les Québécoises et les Québécois Mangent-Ils Mieux? Rapport de l'Enquête Québécoise sur la Nutrition," 1990, both of which measure niacin equivalent intakes, which includes the conversion of tryptophan to niacin. In each case, average consumption is more than triple the estimated average requirement. Canadian intakes are likely lower than American intakes. https://www.ncbi.nlm.nih.gov/books/NBK114320/; and, https://www.ncbi.nlm.nih.gov/books/NBK114304/.

Part V: The Brain-Changing Power of Good Food

Chapter 11. The End of Craving

168 *"delay discounting tasks":* Weller et al., "Obese Women Show Greater Delay Discounting than Healthy-Weight Women"; and Epstein et al., "Women Who Are Motivated to Eat and Discount the Future Are More Obese."

169 *neurodegenerative diseases—and obesity:* Hilbert et al., "Group Cognitive Remediation Therapy for Adults with Obesity Prior to Behavioural Weight Loss Treatment."

176 *The two brain circuits talk to each other:* Castro, Cole, and Berridge, "Lateral Hypothalamus, Nucleus Accumbens, and Ventral Pallidum Roles in Eating and Hunger."

Chapter 13. A Visit to the Old Road

197 *The form of the leaf repeats itself*: Jochen Bockemühl, "Transformations in the Foliage Leaves of Higher Plants," in Seamon and Zajonc, *Goethe's Way of Science*.

197 *a plant is all leaf*: Goethe, Auden, and Mayer, *Italian Journey (1786–1788)*.

197 *Einstein imagined it thus*: Kilmister, *The Environment in Modern Physics: A Study in Relativistic Mechanics*.

198 *"the key to all signs of nature"*: "Morphologie," in Goethe and Richter, *Sämtliche Werke Nach Epochen Seines Schaffens, Münchner Ausgabe*.

Index

addiction, 75–79
  craving/"wanting" and, 76–79
  as euphoric state vs. magnetic pull,
    76–77
  incentive sensitization theory, 77
  negative reinforcement theory of, 76
  obesity and, 77–79
  positive reinforcement theory of, 76
  to sugar/sweet taste, 119–20
  temptation-overload theory of, 77
  withdrawal and, 76
additives, 11, 21–22, *see also* food
    technology
alcohol, *see* wine
alfalfa, as pig feed, 152, 154, 156–57
alginate, 117, 188
American Psychological Association, 77
amphetamines, 69
anal leakage, fake fats and, 122
Anderson, Harvey, 157–58
anti-carb movement, 2–5, 8
anticipatory "liking," 75
Apostles of the Tagliatella, 28, 31
Araujo, Ivan de, 84–86, 87
artificial sweeteners:
  nutritive mismatch and, 87–91, 96,
    118–22, 127, 129
  partial fakeness in, 121–22, 129, 200
  risks of using, 120
  uncertainty and, 118–22, 128
  usefulness of food and, 85–86

Atkins, Robert C., 2, 5
Avicel, 125, 188

B-19 (person in study), 66, 73
bamboo spine, 60
beans:
  in Italian food, 190–91, 194
  niacin in, 18, 19, 150–51
  obesity epidemic and, 151
  soybeans as pig feed, 152–53, 154
behaviorism, 62–66
  behavioral modification and, 8–9
  conditioned stimulus in, 100–103
  drive reduction theory and, 63–66
  Pavlovian responses, 100–101
Berridge, Kent, 70–74, 75, 77–79
Beta-Trim, 125–26
beta-wave therapy, 176
Beyond Meat, 201–2
Biggest Loser, The (TV show), 49–50
Big Gulp, 129
binge-eating disorder:
  craving/"wanting" in, 78, 167–70,
    176–78, 179
  cue-exposure task and, 176–78, 179
  "liking" in treating, 174–76, 186
bitter taste:
  artificial sweeteners and, 121
  denatonium benzoate and, 86
  in detecting poison, 139, 143
  usefulness of food and, 85–86

bliss point, 56–58, 60–61, 92
blood sugar:
   in the carbohydrate-insulin model, 4–7
   nutritive mismatch and, 91, 118
Boakes, Bob, 102–3, 107
body temperature regulation, 37–40, 61,
   67–68
brain:
   addiction and, 75–79
   binge-eating disorder and, 168–69
   body temperature regulation and,
     37–40, 61, 67–68
   cognitive dysfunction in obesity,
     168–69
   dopamine pathways in, 69–75
   expensive tissue hypothesis and, 92–93
   metabolic intelligence and, 40–53, 55,
     61, 66, 68
   negative affect and, 64–65
   nutritional precision and, 11
   nutritive mismatch and, 87–91, 95–97
   omnivore feeding strategy and, 139,
     142–43, 162–64
   opioid receptors and "liking," 74, 77
   pleasure as motivator and, 83–84, 201
   "pleasure center" of, 64–66, 69
   pleasure circuitry in, 140–41
   post-ingestive learning and, 41–42,
     84–85, 87–91
   response frequency and, 65–66
   responses to music, 141–42
   set point and, 40–53
   thrifty gene hypothesis and, 29, 91–92,
     117–18, 199
   uncertainty as grand unifying theory
     of, 108–10
   usefulness of food and, 83–86
Brain: A Journal of Neurology, 83
bread, *see* wheat
breakfast cereal, 96, 158, 159
Brignani, Alice, 188–89
Buffum, Edward Gould, 146
bulimia nervosa, 171–72
bulking, 125
Burger King, 129
butter, 11, 26, 27, 124, 127

button-pushing, 109–10, 187
B vitamins:
   daily consumption in Italy, 161–62
   daily consumption in the US, 159–61,
     161
   in enriching/fortifying food, 21–22,
     150–51, 153, 155–56
   folic acid and pregnancy, 183n
   obesity and, 158–61
   roles in diet, 158–61
   types of, 153

Cabanac, Michel:
   body temperature regulation and,
     37–40, 61, 67–68
   metabolic regulation and, 40–44,
     45–46, 61, 66
   quest for pleasure and, 41–42, 61–68,
     74–75, 84
calories:
   calorie-rich diets and, 92–93
   comparative consumption of, 130
   expensive tissue hypothesis and,
     92–93
   impact of counting, 9
   indirect calorimeter, 88–89
   in "junk food," 29
   nutritive mismatch and, 87–91, 95–97
   post-ingestive learning and, 41–42,
     84–85, 87–91
   on restaurant menus, 9
   sensory tampering and, 117–20
   set point theory and, 47–48
   thrifty gene hypothesis and, 29, 91–92,
     117–18, 199
Canada, obesity in, 157–58
canagliflozin, in diverting sugar, 48
Cannon, Walter, 143
carbohydrate-insulin model, 4–7
carbohydrates:
   in the anti-carb movement, 2–5, 8
   in the carbohydrate-insulin model,
     4–7
   in the carbs-or-fat debate, 1–10, 48
   insulin release and, 139
   in the Italian diet, 25, 27–28, 31, 61

"modified" starches, 126–27, 128, 200
thiamin and appetite for, 160
in the weight-loss process, 1–10, 45, 48
see also grains; pasta; sugar/sweet
taste
carnivores, feeding strategy of, 137–38,
139, 142
carrageenan, 126, 128
Centers for Disease Control, 33
cephalic phase of digestion, 139
Chatonnet, Joseph, 41
cheese:
in Italian food, 26, 27, 28, 31
in the US diet, 26
Chili's, 129
chocolate:
and "liking" to fight craving/
"wanting," 83–84, 87, 174–76,
179–80
pleasure/"reward value" of, 83–84,
87
in treating binge-eating disorder,
174–76
choline, enriching/fortifying food with,
153
Cinnabon, 129
Coca-Cola, 129
cocaine, dopamine levels and, 69
Cold Stone, 129
controlled-feeding experiments, 1–2,
6–7, 45–46
corn:
enriching/fortifying, 22
grits, 20, 22
modern hybrids and, 192–94
"modified" starches from, 126–27, 128,
200
pellagra and, 20, 58, 192–93, 194, 196
as pig feed, 152–53, 154, 156, 159, 192,
193
polenta in the Italian diet, 25, 28,
192–94
vitamin deficiency and, 19–20, 159
craving/"wanting":
addiction and, 76–79
artificial sweeteners and, 120–22

aversion to loss and, 100–103
in binge-eating disorder, 78, 167–70,
176–78, 179
carnivores and, 137–38
combined with "liking," 147–48
cue-exposure task and, 176–78, 179
deliciousness and quality in curing,
174–76
dopamine and, 73–75, 77, 85, 120–22
fake fats and, 123
information exchange with "liking,"
176
"liking" as tool to fight, 173–76
"liking" vs, 74–75, 85
music and, 141–42
obesity and, 112–15
processed foods and, 128–29
separation from "liking," 178
stress and, 175–76
in the thermostat model of eating,
137–38, 140, 142
uncertainty and, 107–10, 112–15
wisdom of the body and, 143–48
Creamfibre 7000, 125, 126, 200
CrystaLean, 125
cue-exposure task, 176–78, 179

daily food diaries, 47–48
dairy products:
ability to digest milk and, 93
in the Italian diet, 26, 27, 28, 31
pellagra and, 18, 19
see also cheese; ice cream; yogurt
Danish food:
lack of enrichment/fortification,
183
taxes on, 183
Dartmouth College, 78
Darwin, Charles, 199
DeKleine, William, 20–21
delay discounting tasks, 168–69
deliciousness, 41–42, 63, 67, 163, 171,
176, 198, see also "liking"
denatonium benzoate, 86
depth psychologists, 62
diabetes, 90–91, 118, 120, 139

diarrhea:
  pellagra and, 16, 19
  pig feed and nutritional deficiency,
    152–53
  sugar alcohols and, 121–22
Dietary Goals for the United States, 2–3
diet foods, 3, 125
Dietz, William, 112–15
dirt eating, 16, 146–47
D-LITE, 125
Doctors Without Borders, 147
"do it by force" approach, 183–86
dopamine, 69–75
  brain lesions and, 70–71
  brain zapping and, 71, 72–73
  craving/"wanting" and, 73–75, 77, 85,
    120–22, *see also* craving/"wanting"
  dopamine-blocking drugs, 70, 73
  dopamine highway and, 74, 88
  "getting stuff" system and, 177
  music and, 141–42
  nutritive mismatch and, 87–91
  Parkinson's disease and, 72
  as the "pleasure chemical," 69–70, 72
  and the thermostat model of eating,
    137–38, 140, 142
  uncertainty and, 107–10
dorsal striatum, 85
Dr. Atkins' Diet Revolution (Atkins), 2, 5
drive reduction theory, 63–66
Duclaux, Roland, 42–43

earth eating, 16, 146–47
economics:
  nature of field, 106
  uncertainty and motivation, 103–10
eggs, pellagra and, 18
Elvehjem, Conrad, 21
emulsifiers, 117, 126–27
energy efficiency:
  expensive tissue hypothesis and,
    92–93
  food storage and, 94–95
enriching/fortifying food, 21–23
  B vitamins in, 21–22, 150–51, 153,
    155–56

countries that do not mandate, 183,
    185, 187–95, 203–4
  nature of, 22, 150
  nutritional information panels and, 96,
    126, 158
  pellagra and, 21–22, 33, 150–51, 183,
    192
  pig feed and, 151–57
  weight gain and, 22–23, 150–61, 183
Enzo (bean farmer), 190–91
erythritol, 129
evolutionary fitness:
  expensive tissue hypothesis and, 92–93
  food storage and, 94–95
  obesity and, 29, 93–94
  taste and, 95, 139, 143
expensive tissue hypothesis, 92–93

fake fats and fat replacers, 122–26,
    128–29, 188, 200
fake meat, 200–202
fast food, *see* junk food
fat receptors, 124–26
fats:
  butter, 11, 26, 27, 124, 127
  in the carbohydrate-insulin model, 4–7
  in the carbs-or-fat debate, 1–10, 48
  Danish tax on foods high in saturated,
    183
  fake fats and fat replacers, 122–26,
    128–29, 188, 200
  fried food and, 26–27, 28, 31–32, 124,
    179–80
  in the Italian diet, 26–27, 31, 162, 194–95
  lard, 194–95
  low-fat diets, 6–7
  olive oil, 26, 31, 32, 191, 194–95
  riboflavin and appetite for, 160
Faust (Goethe), 136
feces, nutrients from, 144
Finnish food, lack of enrichment/
    fortification, 183
finocchi bolognese, 189–90
"fix what's wrong with food" approach,
    11–12, 183–86, 199–203
"flavorings," 127–28, 200

fluorosis (fluoride toxicity), 58–61
folic acid, 183n
food diaries, 47–48
food insecurity, 112–15
food storage, 94–95
food technology, 117–30
    artificial sweeteners, *see* artificial
        sweeteners
    breakfast cereals, 96, 158, 159
    combination systems, 126
    emulsifiers, 117, 126–27
    enriching/fortifying, *see* enriching/
        fortifying food
    fake fats and fat replacers, 122–26,
        128–29, 188, 200
    fake meat, 200–202
    "fix what's wrong with food" approach
        and, 11–12, 183–86, 199–203
    "flavorings," 127–28, 200
    gums, 126–29
    ice cream, 117, 119, 125, 127, 129, 183,
        188
    "liking" approach vs., 191–92
    "modified" starches, 126–27, 128,
        200
    nutritional information panels, 96,
        126, 158
    nutritive mismatch and, 95–97,
        118–22, 129, 130
    origins in the US, 200
    pellagra and, 21–22, 33, 150–51, 183,
        192
    stabilizers, 117, 188
    thickeners, 117, 125
    yogurt, 96, 119, 123–24, 129, 172
French food:
    comparative calorie consumption and,
        130
    lack of enrichment/fortification, 183
    pleasure of eating and, 170–72
Freudians, 62
fried food, 124
    in the Italian diet, 26–27, 28, 31–32
    potato chips, 122, 179–80
    in the US South diet, 26
Frito-Lay, 122

fructose/high-fructose corn syrup,
    160
fruits, 8–9

gambling:
    compared with obesity, 100
    "get money" theory of, 103–4
    loss chasing and, 106–7
    rational choice theory of, 104–6
    uncertainty and, 99–100, 103–7
Gardner, Christopher, 6–7
gas chromatography (GC), 127
Gastellu Etchegorry, Marc, 147
Genugel, 126
Genutine, 126
German food, 170–71
ghrelin, 139
Gladwell, Malcolm, 56
glycogen, 45
goats, human urine and, 144, 162
Goethe, Johann von:
    "doctrine of metamorphosis" and,
        198–99, 202
    exploration through food and,
        202–3
    Faust, 136
    Italian food and, 15–17, 133–36,
        196–200, 201–3
    Italian Journey, 133–35
    pellagra and, 16–17, 196, 199
    as scientist, 196, 199, 202
    The Sorrows of Young Werther, 135
    as statesman, 135–36
    "wholeness" and, 197–98, 201
Goldberger, Joseph, 18–20, 22–23, 51,
    150–51, 196
golden tagliatella standard, 27–28, 31,
    188, 189, 199
grains, 8–9
    breakfast cereal, 96, 158, 159
    storage of, 94
    see also corn; enriching/fortifying
        food; pasta; wheat
grits, 20, 22
groundnuts, pellagra and, 147
gums (food additive), 126–29

Hall, Kevin, 1–2, 4–5, 6, 48, 49–50
Harvard Medical School, 143
heart attack, 8
heart disease, 120
Heath, Robert, 66
heroin:
    addiction to, 76
    "liking" and, 77
high-fiber diets, 92
high-fructose corn syrup/fructose, 160
Hilbert, Anja, 167–80, 186
Hirsch, Jules, 45–46, 47, 51–52
honey, storage of, 94
hookworm, 17
Hungarian food, taxes on, 183
hunger, taste and, 139–40
Hungry Ape Theory of obesity, 29, 91–92,
    117–18, 199

ice cream:
    food technology and, 117, 119, 125,
        127, 129, 183, 188
    in Italy, 27, 31, 188
imitation foods, *see* artificial sweeteners;
    food technology
Impossible Foods, 201–2
incentive sensitization, theory of, 77
India:
    fluorosis research in Karnataka,
        57–61
    pellagra in, 58
indirect calorimeters, 88–89
infection theory of pellagra, 17–18, 19
insulin:
    in the carbohydrate-insulin model,
        4–7
    carbohydrates in releasing, 139
    in cephalic phase of digestion, 139
    nutritive mismatch and insulin
        sensitivity, 90–91, 119
    obesity and, 22–23
insurance hypothesis theory of obesity,
    113–15
iron:
    earth eating and deficiency of,
        146–47

enriching/fortifying food with, 21–22,
    150
isomalt, 121–22
Italian food, 25–33, 187–95
    beans, 190–91, 194
    B vitamins in, 161–62
    carbohydrates in, 25, 27–28, 31, 61,
        see also pasta
    comparative calorie consumption and,
        130
    experience and, 195–99
    fat in, 26–27, 31, 162, 194–95
    finocchi bolognese, 189–90
    fried food in, 26–27, 28, 31–32
    Goethe and, 15–17, 133–36, 196–200,
        201–3
    ice cream/gelato, 27, 31, 188
    junk food and, 31–32
    lardo (Italian delicacy), 26, 162
    "liking" approach and, 163–64,
        173–74, 182, 190–91, 194–95
    Mediterranean diet and, 32
    obesity and, 26, 29–32, 33, 113, 189
    old road (avoidance of enrichment /
        fortification) and, 25–28, 163, 183,
        185, 187–95, 203–4
    olive oil, 31, 194–95
    omnivores and, 162–63
    pasta, *see* pasta
    pellagra and, 15–17, 25–26, 33, 133,
        196, 199
    polenta, 25, 28, 192–94
    popularity of, 29
    sugar/sweet taste in, 27, 31, 161–62
    "thin gene" and, 31
    "traditional" diet vs., 194–95
    wine and, 25–26, 32, 134
Italian Journey (Goethe), 133–35

Japanese food, lack of enrichment/
    fortification, 183
*Journal of the American Medical
    Association*, 9, 19
jowar:
    fluorosis/fluoride toxicity and, 59
    pellagra and, 58

junk food:
  Italian food and, 31–32
  obesity and, 29, 91–92
  taxing, 183, 184–85

Kahneman, Daniel, 103–7
Karnataka, India fluorosis research,
    57–61
Kelco Corporation, 117
ketogenic phase, 2
Keys, Ancel, 32
KFC, 129
Khandare, Arjun, 59–60
kohlrabi, 175
Korean food, lack of enrichment/
    fortification, 183

Lamon, Italy, 190–91
Lancet, 30
lard, 194–95
lardo (Italian delicacy), 26, 162
Learned Brotherhood of the Tortellino,
    28, 31, 61, 202
"liking":
  anticipatory, 75
  authenticity and, 181–82
  as bidirectional, 173–74
  chocolate and, 83–84, 87, 174–76,
    179–80
  combined with craving/"wanting,"
    147–48
  craving/"wanting" vs., 74–75, 85
  deliciousness and, 41–42, 63, 67, 163,
    171, 176, 198
  as a feeling, 181
  food technology vs., 191–92
  French way of eating and, 170–72
  Goethe as the crown prince of, 1
    33–36
  information exchange with "wanting,"
    176
  Italian way of eating and, 163–64,
    173–74, 182, 190–91, 194–95
  music and, 141–42
  omnivores and, 139, 142–43, 163–64
  opioid receptors and, 74, 77

pleasure of eating in obesity treatment,
    170–72, 173–76
  role in quality control, 139, 142–43,
    163–64
  separation from craving/"wanting,"
    178
  taste in, 138, 139–43
  as tool to fight craving/"wanting,"
    173–76
  in treating binge-eating disorder and
    obesity, 174–76, 186
linger, artificial sweeteners and, 121
liver, 20–21
Lorelite, 125
low-carb diets, 5–7, 31
low-fat diets, 6–7
Lycadex, 125–26

maltitol, 121–22
maltodextrin, 87–91, 127, 128, 200
margarine, 125, 127
Masa people (Cameroon and Chad),
    guru walla feeding ritual, 52–53,
    66
Mason, David, 146–47
Mastrangelo, Pino, 195
mayonnaise, 3, 128
McDonald's, 128
McGill University, 64–66, 83
McMaster University, 102
meat:
  Dr. Atkins and, 2
  fake meat, 200–202
  in the Italian diet, 25–26, 31
  pellagra and, 19
  see also protein
Mediterranean diet, 32
metabolic chambers, 2
metabolic syndrome, 120
metabolism:
  mathematical model of, 4–5
  metabolic regulation and, 40–53, 55,
    61, 66, 68
Methocel, 125–26
methylcellulose, 128
Mexican food, taxes on, 183

micronutrients, *see* enriching/fortifying
     food; vitamins
Mitchel, John, 147–48
"modified" starches, 126–27, 128, 200
Moro, Luciano, 193
Moro, Rita, 193–95
Moskowitz, Howard, 56–61, 86
Moss, Michael, 56
motivation:
     pleasure as motivator, 83–84, 201
     uncertain outcome and, 99–112, 182
Mount Vernon Hospital for the Colored
     Insane (Alabama), 17
mouthfeel, 121, 125
music, responses to, 141, 142
Mussolini, Benito, 26

National Institute of Nutrition (India),
     59–60
National Institutes of Health (NIH), 1–2,
     4–5, 160
negative affect, 64–65
negative reinforcement theory of
     addiction, 76
Nettle, Daniel, 93
Neumann, Rudolf Otto, 50
Newcastle University, 93
New York Times Magazine, 3–4
niacin/B3:
     daily consumption in Italy, 162
     daily consumption in the US, 161
     dietary sources of, 18, 19, 20–21,
          25–26, 58, 147, 150–51
     enriching/fortifying food with, 21–22,
          150–51, 153, 155–56
     in pig feed, 153, 155–56
     in preventing fluorosis, 58–61
     in preventing pellagra, 20–22, 25–26,
          58, 150–51, 160
     role in diet, 58–61, 158–60
     sugar consumption and, 160–61, 162
nicotine, addiction to, 76
nicotinic acid, 21
NutraSweet, 125
nutritional information panels, 96, 126,
     158

Nutrition Sciences Initiative (NuSI), 5
nutritive mismatch:
     aversion to loss and, 100–103
     examples of, 96
     fake fats and, 122–26
     processed foods and, 95–97, 118–22,
          129, 130
     sugar/sweet taste and, 87–91, 95–97,
          118–22, 127, 129

obesity, 29–33
     as adaptive response to episodic food
          insufficiency, 112–15
     addiction and, 77–79
     anti-carb movement and, 8
     bean consumption and, 151
     B vitamins and, 158–61
     in Canada, 157–58
     carbohydrate-insulin model and, 4–7
     carbohydrates vs. fats and, 1–10
     cognitive dysfunction and, 168–69
     comorbidities and, 8, 167, 169
     enriching/fortifying food and weight
          gain, 22–23, 33, 157–61, 173
     evolutionary fitness and, 29, 93–94
     food insecurity and, 112–15
     gambling compared with, 100
     Hungry Ape Theory of, 29, 91–92,
          117–18, 199
     imitation food and, 11–12
     insurance hypothesis theory of, 113–15
     in Italy, 26, 29–32, 33, 113, 189
     junk food and, 29, 91–92
     persistent metabolic adaptation and,
          49–53
     pleasure of eating and, 91–92, 170–72
     poverty and, 22–23, 112–15
     risks of, 23
     as a sickness, 11–12, *see also* obesity
          treatment
     stigma regarding, 11–12, 29, 91–92,
          117–18, 199
     theories of weight gain and, 23
     in the US, 22–23, 26, 29–30, 33, 113,
          157–58, 172–73
     as vicious cycle, 167–69

Obesity Belt (US), 23
obesity treatment, 22–23, 167–80
  binge-eating disorder and, 167–70,
    172–73, 174–79, 186
  bulimia nervosa compared with
    obesity and, 172
  controlled-feeding experiments, 1–2,
    6–7, 45–46
  cue-exposure task and, 176–78, 179
  delay discounting tasks in, 168–69
  "liking" replacing craving/"wanting"
    in, 174–76, 186
  persistence in, 169
  stop-signal tasks in, 168, 169–70,
    176
Oikos, 129
Olds, James, 64–66, 69
olestra, 122–23
olive oil, 26, 31, 32, 191, 194–95
Olympic National Park, 144
omnivores:
  dumbing down omnivorous nature,
    182
  feeding strategy of, 142–43, 162–64
  "liking" and quality control, 139,
    142–43, 163–64
  pig farming and, 151–57
  wisdom of the body and, 143–48
opioid receptors, "liking" and, 74, 77

pantothenic acid, in pig feed, 153
parasite theory of pellagra, 18
Parkinson's disease, dopamine and, 72
pasta:
  Apostles of the Tagliatella, 28, 31
  enriching/fortifying, in the US, 22
  Goethe and, 134
  golden tagliatella standard and, 27–28,
    31, 188, 189, 199
  Learned Brotherhood of the Tortellino,
    28, 31, 61, 202
  ragù alla bolognese, 27–28, 188–89,
    195
Pavlov, Ivan, 100–101
peas, pellagra and, 18
Pediatrics, 112

pellagra, 15–22
  diet and, 18–22, 25–26, 33, 58, 147,
    192–94, 196
  enriching/fortifying food to prevent,
    21–22, 33, 150–51, 183, 192
  Goethe and, 16–17, 196, 199
  in India, 58
  infection theory of, 17–18, 19
  in Italy, 15–17, 25–26, 33, 133, 196, 199
  niacin/B3 and, 20–22, 25–26, 58,
    150–51, 160–61
  parasite theory of, 18
  poverty and, 19–22, 25–26, 58
  preventing, 20–22, 25–26
  symptoms of, 15–17
  in the US, 17–23, 33, 196
Pellagra Belt (US), 17, 18, 23
pemmican, 94, 95
persistent metabolic adaptation and,
    49–53
pig farming:
  corn and soybeans in, 152–53, 154,
    156–57, 159, 192, 193
  "drylot" vs. pasturing, 151–57
  feed efficiency in, 153–57
pleasure:
  action at a distance and, 61
  addiction and, 75–79
  behavioral final common path and,
    61–62
  behaviorism and, 62–66
  brain circuitry in, 140–41
  chocolate and, 83–84, 87, 174–76,
    179–80
  dopamine and, 69–75
  as "liking," see "liking"
  measurement problem and, 63, 70–75
  as motivator, 83–84, 201
  obesity viewed as excess of, 91–92,
    170–72
  pleasure centers and, 64–65, 69
  quest for, 41–42, 61–68, 74–75, 84
  self-stimulation and, 65–66, 69
poison, bitter taste in detecting, 139,
    143
polenta, 25, 28, 192–94

Pollan, Michael, 143
positive allosteric modifiers, 122
positive reinforcement theory of
    addiction, 76
post-ingestive learning, 41–42, 84–85,
    87–91
potatoes:
    "modified" starches from, 126–27, 128,
    200
    potato chips, 122, 179–80
    as vitamin C source, 146
poverty:
    fluorosis (fluoride toxicity) and,
    58–61
    food insecurity and, 112–15
    obesity and, 22–23, 112–15
    pellagra and, 19–22, 25–26, 58
    vitamin deficiency and, 19–20, 159
pregnancy:
    folic acid and, 183n
    vitamins and weight gain, 158
processed foods, *see* food technology
protein:
    Dr. Atkins and, 2, 3–4
    fake meat, 200–202
    ghrelin release and, 139
    impact on eating behavior, 161
    whey protein concentrate, 125, 126,
    129, 154
    see also meat
Provenza, Fred, 161
Purdue University, 119, 122–23
pyridoxine, enriching/fortifying food
    with, 153

rabbit meat, 25–26
ragù alla bolognese, 27–28, 188–89, 195
rancid fats, 124
rational choice theory, 104–6
Reese's, 129
refined carbohydrates:
    in the carbohydrate-insulin model, 4
    see also enriching/fortifying food; food
        technology; sugar/sweet taste
restaurant menus, calorie counts on, 9
resting metabolic rate, 49–50

riboflavin:
    daily consumption in Italy, 162
    daily consumption in the US, 161
    enriching/fortifying food with, 21–22,
    150, 153, 155–56
    in pig feed, 153, 155–56
    role in diet, 159, 160
rice:
    enriching/fortifying, in the US, 22
    in the Italian diet, 27, 28
Richter, Curt, 160
Robinson, Terry, 77–79
Rockefeller University Hospital, 45–46,
    47
Rozin, Paul, 143

saccharin, 118, 119–20, 128
Salt Sugar Fat (Moss), 56
salty taste, 56, 92, 124
satiety, 140, 141, 173
Schultz, Wolfram, 83, 107–8
Science, 56, 60–61
Scully, Vin, 99
scurvy, 145–46, 147–48, 149
semistarvation neurosis, 46–47, 50, 67
sensory tampering, 117–20
set point, 40–53
    caloric intake and, 47–48
    changing, 67–68
    persistent metabolic adaptation and,
    49–53
    resting metabolic rate and, 49–50
    semistarvation neurosis and, 46–47,
    50, 67
sexual behavior:
    "curing" homosexuality and (B-19),
    66, 73
    dopamine highway and, 74
    dopamine surges in predicting, 78
    drives and, 63
    elevated dopamine and, 72, 73
    pleasure and, 66, 73
Simplesse, 125, 126, 188
Sims, Ethan, 50–51, 67
skin orgasm, 141, 142
Slendid, 125

Small, Dana:
    nutritive mismatch and, 87–91, 95,
        118, 127
    pleasure as motivator and, 83–84, 201
smoking:
    addiction to nicotine, 76
    dopamine highway and, 74
    Italian diet and, 32
snakes:
    lack of taste sense, 137, 142
    smell and, 137
    and the thermostat model of eating,
        137–38, 140, 142
Society for Neuroscience, 71–72
soda taxes, 183, 184–85
Solka-Floc, 125, 128
Sorrows of Young Werther, The (Goethe),
    135
sour taste, 56–61
soybeans, 152–53, 154
Soylent, 200–201
Spanish food, lack of enrichment/
    fortification, 183
Spector, Herbert, 42–43
spelt bread, 173
stabilizers, 117, 188
starvation:
    internal, in the carbohydrate-insulin
        model, 4
    pellagra as form of, 19
    semistarvation neurosis, 46–47, 50, 67
stealth carbs, 126–27
stevia, 96, 128, 129
St. John's Medical College (Bangalore,
    India), 56–57
stomach:
    importance of taste and, 139–40
    role of, 86
stop-signal tasks, 168, 169–70, 176
storage of food, 94–95
stress:
    artificial sweeteners and response to,
        120–21
    craving/"wanting" and, 175–76
    need for, 163–64
    weight gain and, 23

stroke, 8
sucralose, 85–86, 87, 96, 128, 200
sucrose, 160
sugar alcohols, 121–22, 129, 200
sugar/sweet taste:
    addiction to, 119–20
    artificial sweeteners and, *see* artificial
        sweeteners
    "bliss point" and, 56–58
    canagliflozin in diverting sugar from
        bloodstream, 48
    cross-cultural differences in taste
        preferences and, 56–60
    decline in US sugar consumption, 8
    in the Italian diet, 27, 31, 161–62
    metabolic regulation and, 41–44
    as a metabolic signal, 89–91
    niacin consumption and, 160–61, 162
    nutritive mismatch and, 87–91, 95–97,
        118–22, 127, 129
    pleasure response to, 70–71
    post-ingestive learning and, 41–42,
        84–85, 87–91
    sensory tampering and, 117–20
    sour vs. sweet taste preference and,
        56–61
    "sweet-blindness" and, 84–85, 91
    usefulness of food and, 84–86, 87
superabundant food environment,
    110–11
Swedish food, lack of enrichment/
    fortification, 183
sweet taste, *see* sugar/sweet taste
Swithers, Susie, 119, 122–23

tamarind:
    fluoride entrapment capacity and,
        59–61
    as source of niacin/B3, 58–61
    sour taste preference and, 56–61
tantalizing, 178
Tantalus, 178
taste:
    basic tastes, 124
    bliss point and, 56–58, 60–61, 92
    in the digestion process, 139

taste (*cont.*)
  evolutionary fitness and, 95, 139, 143
  hunger and loss of, 139–40
  lack of taste sense in snakes, 137
  in "liking," 138, 139–43
  reasons for, 138, 139–43
  salty taste, 56, 92, 124
  separation from nutrition, 139–40
  sour taste, 56–61
  taste receptor cells, 124, 139
  see also bitter taste; sugar/sweet taste
Taubes, Gary, 3–5, 6
taxes, on junk food, 183, 184–85
temptation-overload theory of addiction, 77
thermic effect of food, 88–89
thermostat model of eating, 137–38, 140, 142
thiamin:
  daily consumption in Italy, 161
  daily consumption in the US, 159–60
  enriching / fortifying food with, 21–22, 150, 153
  role in diet, 158–60
thickeners, 117, 125
Thinking, Fast and Slow (Kahneman), 104–6
thirst, as a drive, 63
thrifty gene hypothesis, 29, 91–92, 117–18, 199
Tim Hortons, 129
Torbole, Italy, 134, 136
toxins:
  bitter taste in poison detection, 139, 143
  fluorosis (fluoride toxicity), 58–61
  impact on eating behavior, 161
Tulane University, 66
Tversky, Amos, 103–6

uncertainty:
  artificial sweeteners and, 118–22, 128
  aversion to loss and, 99–103, 110–15
  button-pushing and, 109–10, 187
  fake fats and, 122–26
  food insecurity and, 112–15

gambling and, 99–100, 103–7
  as motivator, 99–112, 182
  nutritive mismatch and, 118–22
United States:
  B vitamin consumption in, 159–60, 161
  comparative calorie consumption and, 130
  disordered eating and, 172–73
  "do it by force" approach and, 183–86
  "fix what's wrong with food" approach and, 11–12, 183–86, 199–203, *see also* food technology
  obesity in, 22–23, 26, 29–30, 33, 113, 157–58, 172–73
  pellagra in, 17–23, 33, 196
University of Illinois, pig feed experiments, 152–55, 159
University of Leipzig, 167
University of Stockholm, 110–11
University of Toronto, 157–58
University of Vermont, 50
University of Wisconsin, 21
urine, nutrients in, 144, 162
Utah State University, 161

vegetables, 8–9
  finocchi bolognese, 189–90
  in the Italian diet, 31, 189–90
Venturi, Mariangela, 188–89
vitamins:
  for enriching/fortifying processed foods, 21–22, 33, 150–57
  obesity and, 158–60
  in pig feed, 152–57
  pregnancy and, 158
  vitamin C and scurvy, 145–46, 147–48, 149
  see also B vitamins
vomiting:
  after smoking, 76
  overeating and, 52, 66
  pig feed and nutritional deficiency, 152

Walmart approach to nutrition, 163
"wanting," *see* craving/"wanting"
Washington University, 172

water:
 body temperature regulation and, 37–40, 61, 67–68
 fluoride toxicity and, 58–61
 thirst as a drive and, 63
weight gain:
 addiction and, 77–79
 artificial sweeteners and, 120
 dopamine surges in predicting, 78
 enriched/fortified foods and, 22–23, 150–61, 183
 livestock farming and, 151–57, 161
 in the Masa *guru walla* feeding ritual, 52–53, 66
 metabolic regulation and, 43–44
 persistent metabolic adaptation and, 49–53
 in pregnancy, 158
 set point and, 40–53
 theories of, 23
weight loss:
 carbohydrate-insulin model and, 4–7
 carbohydrates vs. fats and, 1–10, 45, 48
 challenges of, 9–10
 early stages of, 44–45
 life-consuming effort and, 9–10
 metabolic regulation and, 42–43
 obsession with food and, 42, 46
 persistent metabolic adaptation and, 49–53
 physiological changes in, 43, 46–47, 50, 67
 plateau in, 43, 45
 refeeding after, 43–44, 46–47
 semistarvation neurosis and, 46–47, 50, 67
 set point and, 40–53

Werther fever, 135
What the Dog Saw (Gladwell), 56
wheat:
 decline in consumption, 8
 enriching/fortifying white flour, 21–22, 150–51
 in the Italian diet, 25–26, 27
 spelt bread, 173
 storage of grains, 94
 see also pasta
whey protein concentrate, 125, 126, 129, 154
Wilfley, Denise, 172
wine:
 French diet and, 170–71
 German diet and, 170–71
 Italian diet and, 25–26, 32, 134
wisdom of the body, 143–48
 earth eating and, 16, 146–47
 groundnuts and pellagra, 147
 nutrients from feces, 144
 nutrients in urine, 144, 162
 vitamin C and scurvy, 145–46, 147–48, 149
withdrawal, 76
Women's Health Initiative Dietary Modification Trial (1993), 8–9
World Food Travel Association, 29

xylitol, 121–22

Yale University, 9, 84
yeast, 20–21, 25–26
yogurt:
 additives in, 96, 119, 123–24, 129, 172
 desire for plain, 175

About the Author

MARK SCHATZKER is the author of *The Dorito Effect* and *Steak*. He is the writer in residence at the Modern Diet and Physiology Research Center, and his writing has appeared in the *New York Times*, the *Wall Street Journal*, and *Annual Review of Psychology*. He lives in Toronto. For more information, visit www.markschatzker.com.